D1569092

TWO SIDES
OF THE BRAIN

BRAIN LATERALIZATION
EXPLORED

Sid J. Segalowitz

A SPECTRUM BOOK

Prentice-Hall, Inc., Englewood Cliffs, New Jersey 07632

Library of Congress Cataloging in Publication Data

Segalowitz, Sidney J.
  Two sides of the brain.

  "A Spectrum Book."
  Bibliography: p.
  Includes index.
    1. Cerebral dominance.   2. Brain—Localization
of functions.   I. Title.
  QP385.5.S43   1983   612'.825   82-16656
  ISBN 0-13-935304-6
  ISBN 0-13-935296-1 (pbk.)

This book is available at a special discount when ordered in
bulk quantities. Contact Prentice-Hall, Inc., General
Publishing Division, Special Sales, Englewood Cliffs, N.J. 07632.

5 6 7 8 9 i0

ISBN 0-13-935304-6

ISBN 0-13-935296-1 {PBK.}

Prentice-Hall International, Inc., *London*
Prentice-Hall of Australia Pty. Limited, *Sydney*
Prentice-Hall Canada Inc., *Toronto*
Prentice-Hall of India Private Limited, *New Delhi*
Prentice-Hall of Japan, Inc., *Tokyo*
Prentice-Hall of Southeast Asia Pte. Ltd., *Singapore*
Whitehall Books Limited, *Wellington, New Zealand*
Editora Prentice-Hall do Brasil Ltda., *Rio de Janeiro*

Contents

Preface   vi

Acknowledgements   viii

Introduction   1

1   An historical overview   4

PART ONE—EVIDENCE
FROM THE CLINIC   17

2   Intellectual disorders from unilateral
    brain damage   19

3   Separating the left brain
    from the right brain   45

PART TWO—HEMISPHERE
ASYMMETRIES IN NORMALS   61

4   Ways of measuring brain lateralization   63

082952

5 Lateralization for language functions 85

6 Nonlinguistic functions 97

PART THREE—DEVELOPMENTAL ISSUES 107

7 Brain lateralization in the developing child 109

8 The evolution of lateralization 125

PART FOUR—INDIVIDUAL
DIFFERENCES 139

9 Is everyone lateralized the same? 141

10 Are some less lateralized than others? 158

11 Are there left and right hemisphere
personalities? 173

PART FIVE—IMPLICATIONS OF
BRAIN LATERALIZATION
FOR HUMAN BEHAVIOR 185

12 Theories of brain lateralization: what
underlies hemisphere asymmetries? 187

13 Is brain lateralization related
to specific mental conditions? 200

14 Hemisphere asymmetries in psychodynamic
processes 212

**PART SIX—SOME ISSUES
FOR THE FUTURE**   223

15   **When is an asymmetry not an asymmetry?**   225

16   **Mapping the mind onto the brain**   234

     Glossary   239

     References   244

     Index   280

Preface

The question of how the brain corresponds to the mind has intrigued scientists and nonscientists for centuries. The finding that the two hemispheres that comprise the bulk of the brain correspond to different aspects of the mind has brought this aspect of the brain sciences to popular attention. Indeed, the importance of this work has been underscored by the awarding of the Nobel prize to Roger Sperry for his seminal work in this field. Despite, or perhaps because of, the simplicity of the left-right dichotomy, the field of brain lateralization has developed at an accelerating pace over the past two decades, involving now thousands of research reports. This rapid growth in interest and research has drawn the attention of the public at large, not to mention psychologists, neurologists, educators, philosophers, historians, artists and other specialists whose business it is to explore the nature of the human mind. This widespread interest, especially by those not involved in the scientific study of lateralization, has led to considerable enthusiasm (and over-enthusiasm) about what the left-right dichotomy can explain.

I have intended, in this book, to present an overview of this field of research, with enough detail to allow the reader to gain some

PREFACE / vii

perspective on how the research is done. At the same time, I have tried to keep the presentation concise and readable, having included references to original research reports or more technical reviews for those interested in following up on certain aspects. The overall purpose of writing this book was to present a text that would discuss the uses of the left-right distinction between the brain hemispheres, as well as give some perspective on the limitations of the construct. This book is addressed to an audience with no previous special knowledge of either physiology or psychology.

Those readers with some background in brain lateralization may find the breadth of coverage useful. I have purposely left some of the philosophical and methodological issues for the end since it would be appropriate for readers to have some background before dealing with paradigmatic problems. Those with some knowledge of neuropsychology or lateralization may want to read Part VI first.

I have a great many people to thank for their help and encouragement on this project over the past two years. Of the many colleagues with whom I have had many invaluable discussions bearing directly and indirectly on the material in this book, I would especially like to thank Phil Bryden and John Benjafield. As well, I am very grateful to the informal army of constructively critical reviewers I am glad to count as friends· Jack Adams-Webber, Linda Bebout, Linda Bramble, Henri Cohen, Jane Dywan, Howard Gardner, Andrew Kertesz, Keith McGowan, Julie Morgan, Samuel Randor, Norm Segalowitz, Linda Siegel, Harry Whitaker, and members of the Psychology 490 class of Brock University of 1981-82. I am also very grateful to Jane Dywan for a number of the handdrawn figures in the book, to Norm Segalowitz for the sound spectographs given in Chapter 12, and to Sandra Witelson for the stimuli reproduced in Figure 4.5. Some of my own research reported here was funded in part by grants from the Natural Science and Engineering Research Council and the Social Science and Humanities Research Council of Canada. I am also very grateful to the Psychology Department of the University of Waterloo for the support they showed me while on leave there during 1980-81, and for the use of the wonderful word processor at that university.

S.J.S.
Brock University
St. Catharines, Ontario

Acknowledgements

Excerpt from M.S. Gazzaniga is used by permission of Plenum Publishing Corporation and the author.

Excerpt from K.M. Heilman and R.T. Watson, "The Neglect Syndrome—a Unilateral Defect of the Orienting Response", in S.R. Harnad, R.W. Doty, L. Goldstein, J. Jaynes & G. Krauthamer, eds., *Lateralization in the Nervous System.*

Wilder Penfield and Lamar Roberts, *Speech and Brain Mechanisms.* Copyright 1959 by Princeton University Press. Figure 1.3 and Table 2.2 reprinted by permission of Princeton University Press.

Figure 2.2 from Kertesz, Lesk, and McCabe (1977), Isotope localization of infarcts in aphasia. *Archives of Neurology, 34*, 590–601. Copyright 1977 American Medical Association. Reprinted by permission of the publisher and the author.

Figure 2.3 from D. Kimura, Acquisition of a motor skill after left-hemisphere damage. *Brain,* Vol. 100 (3), 1977, 527–542. Reprinted by permission.

Figure 4.1 from Vanderplas and Garvin, "The association value of random shapes." *Journal of Experimental Psychology,* 57, 147–154. Copyright 1959 by the American Psychological Association. Reprinted by permission of the publisher and the author.

Figure 4.4 from Ley and Bryden (1979), Hemispheric differences in processing emotions and faces. *Brain and Language,* 7, 127–138. Reprinted by permission of Academic Press and the author.

Figure 4.9 from David H. Ingvar. Functional landscapes of the dominant hemisphere, *Brain Research, 107* (1976), page 188, Figure 3. Reprinted by permission from Elsevier Biomedical Press.

Figure 7.3 from Porac, Coren, and Duncan (1980), Life-span trends in laterality. Journal of Gerontology, *35,* 715–721. Reprinted by permission of *The Gerontologist/The Journal of Gerontology.*

Tables 9.1 and 9.4 from Rasmussen and Milner, The Role of Early Left-Brain Injury in Determining Lateralization of Cerebral Speech Functions. Vol. 299, *Annals of the New York Academy of Sciences,* 1977. Reprinted by permission of the publisher and authors.

Figure 13.1 from Selfe (1977), *Nadia: a case of extraordinary drawing ability in an autistic child.* Copyright Academic Press Inc. (London) Ltd. Reprinted by permission.

Figure 13.2 from Frumkin, Ripley, and Cox. Changes in cerebral hemispheric lateralization with hypnosis. *Biological Psychiatry, 13,* 1978, 741–750. Reprinted by permission of Plenum Publishing Corporation.

Introduction

When a pin-up was flashed without warning to the right
hemisphere of Case II, amongst a series of more routine stimuli,
she first said, upon being asked by the examiner, that she saw
nothing, but then broke into a hearty grin and chuckle. When
queried as to what was funny, she said that she didn't know, that
the "machine was funny, or something."
Case I would sometimes find himself pulling his pants down
with one hand and pulling them up with the other. Once he
grabbed his wife with his left hand and shook her violently, while with
the right trying to come to his wife's aid. . . .

GAZZANIGA (1970)

The patient was a right-handed, middle-aged teacher who had
previously enjoyed excellent health. Although the patient denied
having any difficulties, . . . when asked to read, he read only those
words found on the right side of the page. When words like
toothpick and *baseball* were presented to him, he read *pick* and
ball. He was able to recognize faces. However, when he dressed, he
did not attempt to put on the left side of his clothing. He shaved
only the right side of his face. When asked to draw a daisy, he
drew petals only on the right side. When asked to bisect a line he
would quarter it (three quarters on the left and one quarter on the

right). When asked to cross out lines on a page, he would cross out
only those lines on the right side of the page. When eating, he
would eat food only from the right side of the plate.
HEILMAN & WATSON (1977)

This book is an introduction to the field of brain lateralization, the study of left-right asymmetries in brain functioning. For a long time, the existence of such asymmetries has been recognized and used as a valuable clinical tool, but until recently there was not much detailed exploration of the special activities and abilities of each half of the brain. However, toward the end of the 1960s the atmosphere changed. The slow, rather academic field of study was infused with tremendous enthusiasm and energy sparked by two events. The first was a rising general interest in the biological foundations of behavior, the question of what comprises the biological basis for our very human activities, such as language. The second was much more specific: Detailed studies were made of some special patients (such as in the first two examples above), patients who for medical reasons had had the connections between the two halves of their brains severed. These "split-brain" patients, as they came to be known, could be shown to have two somewhat independently functioning brains and two minds that were not identical in abilities, or desires!

These events captured the imagination of many, scientists and nonscientists alike. Here was an obvious, concrete example of the correspondence between body and mind, between the brain as a biological entity and the mind as a collection of ideas, abilities, needs, and thoughts. This alone should have been enough to spark interest, as the mind/body problem had been debated actively for thousands of years without much data to work with on the "body" half of the formula (i.e. the brain).

However, these studies raised other fascinating issues: Do all of us have two minds within us that struggle for expression? Do the two halves of the brain house different personalities that make up our complex human psyches? Is this why people are so complex? Can studies of the differences between the two halves of the brain help us discover how the human brain, and therefore presumably the human mind, divides up the world? Can they show us how people think about their surroundings, what distinctions they make, to help us decide among the myriad theories that exist?

From these many perspectives, the discovery of lateral asymmetries in the brain raises hopes and insights. Of course as with all new, promising discoveries, much of the speculation about brain lateralization goes far beyond the available data. To support them, one needs more faith than scientific acumen. And, as usual, the issues have turned out to be more complicated than first expected, but nonetheless fascinating. In this book, we will explore the foundation for the hopes and excitement surrounding the field with the closest we can come to sober enthusiasm.

Plan of the Book

We will try to cover as many aspects of brain lateralization as possible, beginning with evidence from the neuropsychology clinic, including work with the split-brain patient. The case studies from the clinic have provided us with many suggestions about how to pose correct questions about mind-brain correlates. But rather than wait for nature or fate to provide us with just the right clinical cases, many scientists have devised ways of investigating brain functions in volunteer normals (without harming them, of course). In Part II, we will review these methods, and explore the differences found between the hemispheres in language functions and other intellectual and perceptual skills.

In Part III, we turn to developmental issues: What is the course of brain lateralization in the growing child and in evolution, comparing species? Part IV is devoted to individual differences. We examine the extent to which the generalizations made so far are valid for all people. Besides the possibility of personality having some effect on brain lateralization, there are also differences that complicate the picture between the sexes and between left- and right-handed people.

Part V is devoted to applications to human behavior outside the laboratory. First, a summary of approaches to the duality of the brain will be given, and then the attempts to extrapolate beyond the laboratory will be examined critically. The last section, Part VI, concerns some philosophical issues raised by research of this kind. No scientific research is purely the gathering of data. Rather, it is also a reflection of the assumptions of the researcher. Some of these assumptions, unquestioned in the past for the sake of simplicity, must now be addressed if we are to continue the growing understanding of the brain's activity.

chapter one

An historical overview

If I forget thee, O Jerusalem, let my right hand
forget her cunning;
If I do not remember thee, let my tongue cleave
to the roof of my mouth.
Psalm 137

Was the biblical linking of control over the right hand and the ability
to speak a medical insight or a reflection of the two most valued
skills? The medical aspect is this: Brain damage that leads to
paralysis of the right side often incapacitates speech as well because
both are controlled by the left side of the brain.

Nowadays, we take for granted that the brain is intimately
related to behavior and thinking. Yet we cling to remnants of an
earlier age, like the notion of the soul residing in the heart. As Shakespeare asked, "Tell me where is fancie bred/Or in the heart, or in the
head."[1] It was not until relatively recently, in the early 1800s, that the
brain itself and its surface grey matter, the part of the brain we
consider crucial for higher human thoughts, began to be accorded the

4

importance they deserve. Before this time, attempts to locate emotion, memory, or reason centered on the fluid-filled cavities in the brain or even in abdominal sections of the body.[2]

Some Basic Neurophysiology

Before we trace the development of the notion that the two sides of the brain serve different functions, we should outline the basic structures involved. The human brain contains about 12 billion *neurons*, which are the cells that fire electrical impulses, and many more other cells that serve various other functions in the brain. Each neuron (see Figure 1.1) consists of (1) one *cell body* containing genetic material that is the "headquarters" for the cell; (2) a number of *dendrites* that

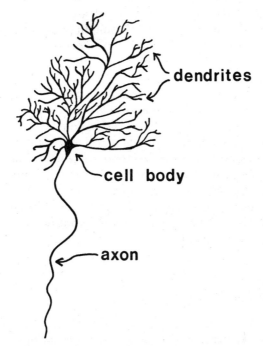

FIGURE 1.1. A number of different types of neurons exist in the brain. Each has a cell body (or nucleus) and quite a number of extending parts, some carrying signals towards the cell body, some carrying impulses to other cells.

transmit incoming impulses to the cell body from other cells; and (3) an *axon* that transmits the neuron's own firing to other cells. When a cell receives enough incoming impulses, it fires, and so the chain continues. However, the chain is exceedingly complex because each neuron has an average 10,000 dendrites and one long axon that splits toward the end into a number of terminals.

Each neuron is much too small to be seen without a microscope, but in masses of tens of millions, they form recognizable patterns. The large mass of brain tissue is called the *cerebrum*. The cerebrum is divided into two similar halves, called the *cerebral hemispheres*. The cell bodies on the surface form a layer called the *cerebral cortex*, which is often called grey matter because of its color. Under this mantle of only a few millimeters in thickness are billions of axons, the connecting fibers, called the white matter. The axons are white due to specialized cells that form a sheath around each one. It is generally accepted that more advanced thought processes depend on the health of the cortex, although *subcortical* neurons (those with their cell bodies in clusters below the cortex) are necessary for, and very involved in, all aspects of behavior.

For convenience, each cerebral hemisphere is divided into four main areas: the *frontal lobe*, the *parietal lobe*, the *temporal lobe* and the *occipital lobe* (see Figure 1.2). The divisions between the lobes are marked by the convolutions, or foldings of the cortex. These foldings are made necessary by the relative lack of space in the head cavity. The two hemispheres are joined by several bundles of connecting fibers, linking specific spots in the cortex of one hemisphere with the analogous spot in the cortex on the other side. The largest of these bundles by far is the *corpus callosum*, about which we will have much to say in this book.

The Beginnings of Neuropsychology

Discovery of the differences between the left and right cerebral hemispheres is just one part of the story of neuropsychology, the goal of which is to better understand how the brain and mind are related. A principal theme in this search concerns the nature of the

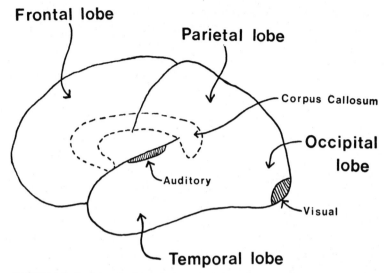

FIGURE 1.2. Each cerebral hemisphere is divided for convenience into 4 lobes. Portrayed here is the left hemisphere of someone facing to the left. Also indicated are the primary projection areas for visual and auditory stimulation, and the corpus callosum, which is the main commissure connecting the two hemispheres.

representation of the mind in the brain. Is the mind (or some part of the mind) represented in the brain as a whole, or can the mind be divided into psychological units located in specific spots? The way the *holist* and the *localizationist* positions have alternated in popularity leads one to suspect that there are grains of truth in both positions. We shall see that how one phrases the question determines to a large extent the answer one gets on this issue.

The search for an understanding of the brain's functioning led, in the last century, to a fascination with the convolutions of the cortex. One reason is that people started to notice that the pattern is regular, unlike other anatomical folds such as in the intestines. This interest increased with the popularity of *phrenology*, which can best be described as a movement to link physiology and psychology. Reasoning that specific psychological traits should reside in specific brain locations, Franz Gall (1758–1828) and his enthusiastic student Johann Spurzheim (1776–1832) suggested that the shape of the skull would reflect the relative strength or weakness of the traits residing below. As it became the rage to measure everyone's head, the scientific respectability of the notion waned. However, in its wake, phrenology left new interest in the idea that psychological traits could be localized in a particular brain region, specifically in the convolutions on the surface of the brain.

Scientific attempts to disprove the extreme statements about localizing specific psychological traits in specific centers followed. This was done by demonstrating that the loss of one specific area of brain tissue often does not alter an animal's behavior compared to loss of another area. Yet even in these studies there were some behavioral disturbances resulting from differences in the location of the damage, and the medical elite of Europe was ready in the latter half of the 1800s to swing towards the localization hypothesis. In 1861, Paul Broca, the noted French surgeon and anthropologist, presented two cases of patients diagnosed independently as having a loss of speech. Both of them had suffered damage to the left frontal part of the brain (see Figure 1.3). Their right hemispheres were intact. Soon afterwards, Broca proclaimed a rule that in right-handers, speech is represented in the left side of the brain, and that in left-handers it is in the other side. Shortly after this in 1870, the German physiologists, Gustav Theodor Fritsch and Edward Hitzig reported that electrically stimulating one side of a dog's brain produces movement in the opposite half of the body. In short order, they and others developed maps of brain functions, much as the phrenologists had done, but on a more sound scientific basis.[3] The phrenologists had been guessing from both ends of the mind-brain link, not being able to be sure either about the psychological traits (should one look for a "love of children" center in the brain or simply a "love" center?) or the locations on the skull. The localizationists, on the other hand, were often more careful about the psychological trait being investigated, by asking specific questions about, say, speech production as distinct from comprehension, and then testing their notions experimentally.

FIGURE 1.3. The photograph is of a real brain with various regions marked: the anterior and posterior language regions of the left hemisphere. The schematic shows the pattern of movement representations. From Penfield & Roberts (1959). Reprinted by permission.

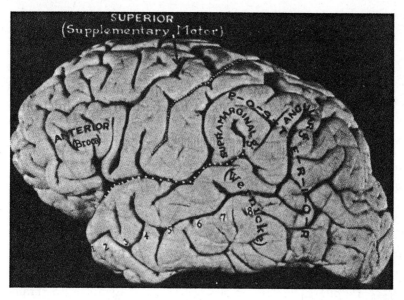

SUPERIOR
(Supplementary, Motor)

ANTERIOR
(Broca)

SUPRAMARGINAL

ANGULAR

POSTERIOR
(Wernicke)

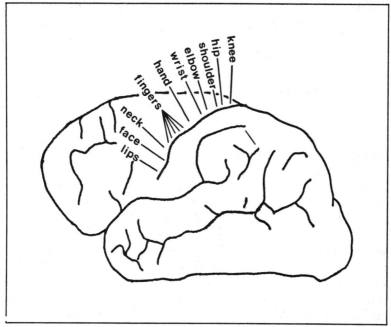

knee
hip
shoulder
elbow
wrist
hand
fingers
neck
face
lips

Are the Two Hemispheres Physically Identical?

Until the middle of the last century, the notion of localization of function in the brain was considered radical enough without the postulation of differences between the hemispheres. However, Broca's presentations in 1861 pointed the way to the left-sided representation for language. At this time, John Hughlings Jackson in England suggested that the functions of the right hemisphere would one day be shown to complement the linguistic abilities of the left.[4] In 1874, the German neurologist Carl Wernicke described a type of language loss different from Broca's cases, involving damage to the left hemisphere but in a different spot (see Figure 1.3). In Broca's cases, the patients seemed to lack the ability to coordinate the movements necessary for speech and usually had a right-sided paralysis, but they could comprehend satisfactorily. In Wernicke's case, the loss was of the meaning of the words, and there was no loss of movement.

Despite such clinical observations, the asymmetry of brain functioning was resisted for one main reason: If the two sides serve such radically different functions, why do the two hemispheres *look* so similar? One would expect functional differences to be paralleled by some physical differences, and yet if any anatomical differences exist, they are not easily detectable. First, the two hemispheres are the same overall length. Individual variation is found, but in terms of total length, weight or volume, there is no consistent asymmetry. Within each hemisphere, however, there appear to be some interesting consistent differences between the left and right sides. For example, the *Sylvian fissure*, a major landmark on the cortex, is usually longer on the left side and is pointed more upwards on the right.[5] This means that certain areas on the left temporal lobe associated with language functions are larger than the similarly located areas on the right (called *homologous* areas).[6] Of course, some other areas must be greater on the right than on the left in order to equalize the hemispheres in overall size. Whether or not these asymmetries in size are related to differences in function is still an open question. The physical asymmetries are subtle, the functional differences are great. It is clear that if there is a relationship between size of brain area and type of skill, it is not a simple one.

Can the Mind
Be Reduced to the Brain?

A constant argument against the localizationist position is the subjective feeling we have about the unity of our experience. We see the world through one "mind's eye," we have one soul apiece.[7] How could it be that the brain is a grouping of separate parts if the mind is an integrated whole? This concern with keeping some unity of the senses has led to a migration of the brain site said to be responsible for it. In ancient times, some placed the unifying organ in one of the cavities of the brain, others in the *rete mirabile* (a network of vessels placed in the front of oxen's heads that unfortunately doesn't exist in humans). Descartes suggested the *pineal gland* as the seat of the soul (or at least the point of interaction with the body) and the director of mental functions because it is not a double structure. The most recent allocation for the integrating and decision-making structure (no longer called the soul) is the "association areas" of the brain. These areas are not involved directly in receiving sensations from the world, but rather in integrating them. This concern with finding a brain location where all the various experiences come together is a reflection of how uncomfortable people are with biological reductionism—the attempt to relate (or perhaps, reduce) the functions of mind to biological structures. When the mind is divided into various functions such as perception, memory, language, and so on, people often feel that there must be some overall organizer, some integrating, responsible component. The modern dilemma is that we have enough information now to see the naivete of the notion of one command center controlling each person's free will—essentially another little person in the head—yet we have no models for accounting for behavior without one. The notion of a "highest" center in the brain is a welcome feudal concept, but unfortunately is too simple for reality. There is no command center, but rather a network of interacting brain structures. The interactions in the brain and the feedback loops are so complex that on logical grounds alone there cannot be a command center. Rather, there is a system that makes decisions as a whole.[8] Yet this is not an impediment to postulating subsystems within the brain, as modern neuropsychology is now finding.

Why Is Correlating Brain Structures to Functions of Mind so Difficult?

The task of neuropsychology is ambitious indeed. In attempting to find links between brain activity and the functions of the mind, we must appreciate that we have a problem similar to the brain teasers in the newspaper, but magnified a thousand fold. In a brain teaser, we are given a few facts and must discover many more by good guesswork and careful reasoning. In correlating mind and brain, we have very few facts, a few "equations" and very many unknowns.[9] First of all, the functions of mind are not obvious and there seem to be almost as many theories of what the mind is about as there are psychologists. As well, unfortunately, it is not at all obvious what the appropriate unit of brain activity should be. Should we examine single neurons, groups of neurons, systems of neurons not adjacent but linked nevertheless, and so on. To complicate matters further, it is not at all obvious which functions of mind should be correlated with brain structures and which should be ignored. Presumably, chess playing or skateboard riding are too complex to be related directly to one brain structure each, whereas matching visually two items may be a simple enough function. This difficulty of finding the correct psychological level was a basic problem the phrenologists had (see Figure 1.4). Similarly, how much dividing up of the brain is appropriate? Clearly, this could get out of hand (see Figure 1.5). Other problems complicate the matter further, such as that every person has a unique personality and a unique brain and that single brain systems have many functions simultaneously. That any progress has been made at all is a tribute to human ingenuity, intuition, and doggedness.

Brain lateralization, as a field, has grown remarkably faster than other areas of neuropsychology, largely because one important difficulty was removed. The unit of brain function is not of primary concern, but rather only the side on which the activity occurs is important. This simplifies matters considerably. In Part I, we will see how clinical cases of brain damage have given us much information

---

FIGURE 1.4. The phrenologists were concerned with finding the locations in the brain where psychological faculties are represented. From Clarke & Dewhurst (1972). Reprinted by permission.

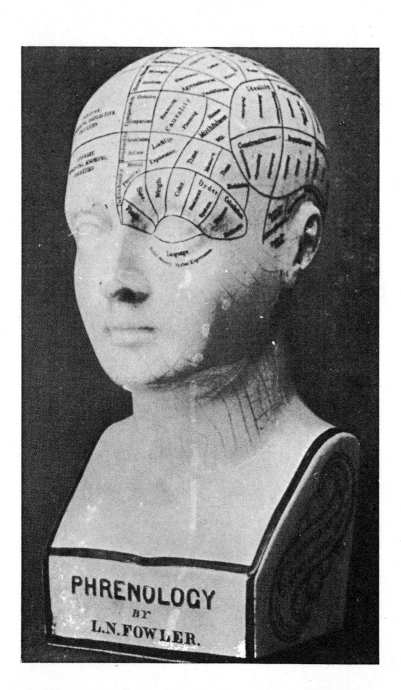

PHRENOLOGY
BY
L.N. FOWLER.

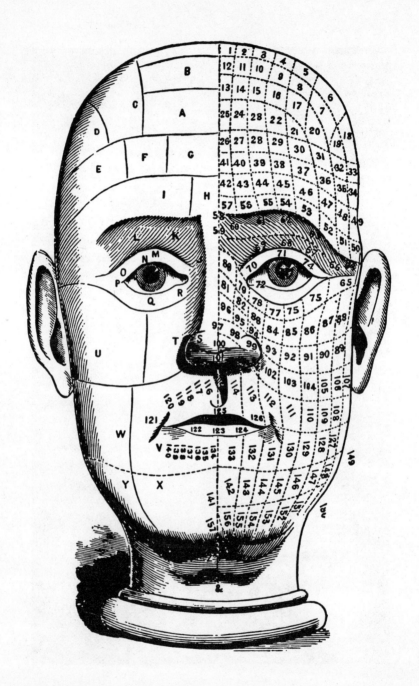

about the lateralization of psychological functions, while we remain ignorant to a large extent about the functioning at the more detailed within-hemisphere level.

NOTES

1. Merchant of Venice, Act III, Scene ii, 64.
2. A well-illustrated and readable history of brain function extending back to ancient times is presented by Clarke & Dewhurst (1972).
3. See Krech (1962) for a summary of the events and controversies of this period.
4. Jackson (originally published in the *Medical Press and Circular* in 1874, but reprinted in 1915 in *Brain*; also reprinted in Taylor, 1932) showed incredible insight when we consider the relatively small amount of data he had to work from. Many of his statements, which could better be described as predictions of what would be found later, are now being supported.
5. Rubens (1977), Geschwind & Levitsky (1968).
6. See Witelson (1977b, 1980) for reviews.
7. Admittedly, the soul and the mind need not refer to the same thing, a point Bogen (1969) uses to argue for a multiple-component mind. However, from an experimental point of view, the two are usually considered the same.
8. A fascinating discussion of this issue is presented in *Brain and Behavioral Sciences*, Volume 1, 1978. See especially Andreae (1978).
9. See Uttal (1978, chapter 5) and Glassman (1978) for discussions on this point.

FIGURE 1.5. The enthusiasm for finding brain centers for specific faculties of mind sometimes led to absurd maps. From Clarke & Dewhurst (1972). Reprinted by permission.

part one

EVIDENCE FROM THE CLINIC

Although it was not always clear from laboratory studies that specific intellectual functions could be localized in the brain, clinicians have known better from practical experience. A patient would often arrive with a fairly specific loss of function through brain damage, such as of reading, or of writing, or the ability to recognize faces. The fact that an ability can be so selectively impaired naturally leads one to assume that the skill in question must have been dependent on some specific portion of the brain, and that this portion was the damaged part. The difficulty lies in making consistent and plausible connections between functions and brain areas. The fact that neurological disorders can be so specific is at the same time both a boon and a bane to the search for neuropsychological order. There are enough patterns found in the symptoms to spur the search. But the range of patterns becomes a disadvantage. It seems at first glance that every patient is unique (which is true inasmuch as every person is unique). How can order be found when there are so many patterns of symptoms? Add to this the relatively elementary state of physiological analysis of the brain until fairly recently, and one can see why the task of neuropsychology at times becomes fanciful theorizing rather than empirical study.

Of course there were hints. For example, there were isolated but clear cases of left-sided brain damage causing language loss. But the variation in symptoms and in the types of brain damage was tremendous. We have seen how, after several false starts, the current notions of neuropsychology took shape in the last half of the nineteenth century. After the basic work of Broca, Wernicke, and Fritsch and Hitzig, the idea of localization of function was finally respectable, and even included the foundations of hemisphere asymmetries. Most important, these developments allowed researchers to make predictions about brain-behavior relationships, especially hemispheric differences, which increased the attention paid to the quest. There was a better idea of what to look for, and researchers were no longer forced to rely solely on extensive experience and clinical acumen to intuit the relationships, and so the evidence began pouring in. Cases of disorders of movement and functions of the senses were most clear. But also, there naturally was interest in intellectual functions, often of a subtle kind, associated with specific brain damage.

Traditionally, these disorders were divided into three sub-groups: disturbances of language functions, called aphasias; disturbances in the organization of movements, called apraxias; and disturbances of knowledge, called agnosias. Chapter 2 provides an overview of these syndromes and how they reflect the differences in the functioning of the right and left sides of the brain. Chapter 3 gives an overview of a fairly new clinical case: The split-brain patient whose two halves are literally separated, and who, at times, seems to have two, somewhat different minds.

chapter two

Intellectual disorders from unilateral brain damage: aphasia, apraxia, and agnosia

Many disturbing yet fascinating disorders can result from brain damage, producing distortions in a person's intellect or personality. Not all of them, of course, are due to *unilateral* damage, that is, a trauma to only one side of the brain. Some disorders only arise when both sides are affected. For example, despite the apparent superiority of the right hemisphere in recognizing faces (see Chapter 6), a complete loss of this ability requires simultaneous damage to both sides in specific regions. A person with this problem is unable to recognize people well known to him, including close relatives. Once the visitor begins to speak, recognition of the voice allows a somewhat normal interaction, or the patient may have to relearn that father has a moustache and use this cue for recognition. Despite this dramatic symptom (called *prosopagnosia* or *facial agnosia*), there is no other obvious loss in visual skill. These patients can easily and accurately describe visual objects, including faces. It is only the recognition of familiar faces that the patient has difficulty with.[1]

For a syndrome to be deemed due to unilateral damage, it must be shown that the symptoms are associated with damage to one side. Exceptions to this condition must be explainable. For example, such exceptions arise in cases of brain damage early in life, which can cause a reorganization of how skills are represented in the brain. Of course, it is not always clear whether the particular patient being examined is a justified exception or whether we have our syndrome wrong. Such is the frustration of neuropsychology!

Neuropsychologists have noticed, however, a number of recurrent patterns that suggest an association between side of damage and type of symptom. As the field has progressed, more and more cases have been collected, and now we can evaluate the pattern in hundreds of individuals. The most serious complaints become, of course, the best studied ones. These interfere dramatically with the person's ability to function in ordinary life and so have merited the most attention. They are disorders of language and communication (aphasia), disorders of skilled movement (apraxia), and disorders of recognition and knowledge (agnosia). In this chapter, discussion will be confined as much as possible to examples that relate to unilateral damage, that is, ones that aid in our understanding of lateralization in the brain. More complete summaries of these syndromes are available elsewhere.[2]

Double Dissociation.   Distinguishing symptoms is not always easy. How can we tell whether or not one particular symptom is just a more severe form of another? The technique used is called *double dissociation*: if patients can be found showing one symptom but not a second, while other patients show the second but not the first, then we say that the two are dissociated and represent different syndromes. For example, as is described in the next section, producing, comprehending, and repeating speech are dissociated.

Aphasia

The best-founded asymmetric function of the brain is language. Although language disturbances can come in a variety of forms, they almost invariably involve the left hemisphere. It is estimated that at least 95% of all people conform to this pattern of left dominance for language. Almost all exceptions are either left-handers or are right-handers who have suffered some form of brain disease, such as epilepsy, early in life. But, even the majority in these groups are left dominant for language (see Chapter 9).

A number of systems have been proposed to account for the variety of language disorders. For historical reasons, the names of the syndromes vary, but the symptoms are generally agreed upon. To illustrate the range, we will very briefly review them with a focus on the production of, the comprehension of, and the ability to repeat speech. First consider comprehension and production. Although we rarely see a disorder of one exclusively with the other completely intact, some aphasics are affected more in their comprehension and others more in their production. A production deficit is characterized by halting speech, as in this case where the patient explains that he has a dentist appointment.

> Ah . . . Monday . . . ah, Dad and P.H. (referring to himself by his full name) and Dad . . . hospital. Two . . . ah, doctors . . . , and ah . . . thirty minutes . . . and yes . . . ah . . . hospital. And, er Wednesday . . . nine o'clock. And er Thursday, ten o'clock . . . doctors. Two doctors . . . and ah . . . teeth. Yeah, . . . , fine.[3]

This syndrome is generally called *Broca's aphasia*, although it is also associated with other names such as *motor aphasia* and *frontal* or *anterior aphasia*. It seems as if putting words together has become a great chore for the patient even though there is nothing physically wrong with his lips and tongue. It appears that the patient tries to use as few words as possible—mainly nouns, verbs and adjectives. Comprehension is relatively well preserved in Broca's aphasia. However, the characterization of Broca's aphasia as only one of expression is rather simplistic since the difficulty extends to writing. As well, such patients have difficulty with some grammatical judgments.[4]

In contrast to this, *Wernicke's aphasia* refers to a loss primarily in comprehension, producing a veritable word salad, as in this example.

> I feel very well. My hearing, writing been doing well, things that I couldn't hear from. In other words, I used to be able to work cigarettes I didn't know how . . . This year, the last three years, or perhaps a little more, I didn't know how to do me any able to.

Wernicke's aphasia includes a definite disorder of meaning. In this case, it is as if the grammar can be used somewhat independently of the thought, so of course nonsense is produced. However, such patients do not seem to be aware of the lack of sense they are making, or at least, their speech is fluent, comfortable, and apparently free of frustration. It seems that all combinations of disruption of production, comprehension, and repetition have been noted among aphasics, and labelled as in Table 2.1. For example, Broca's and Wernicke's aphasics have great difficulty repeating phrases to an examiner, each for different reasons. But there is another, less common, type of aphasia, where there is no difficulty in repetition or in comprehension, but only in producing new sentences. This syndrome, called *transcortical motor* or *dynamic aphasia*, seems to involve a difficulty in planning. Alexandr Luria describes the problem as involving the putting together of phrases. The patient has no difficulty with stereotyped, short sentences, but when a new integrated series is required, as in telling a new story, the patient cannot get started. One therapy, suggested by Luria, involves providing an external structure for the patient to lean on, such as a row of pieces of paper. The patient can get started if he coincides his first phrase with touching the first piece of paper, the next phrase with the next one, and so on.[5]

Similarly, another syndrome involves preserved repetition and production (albeit with many semantic substitutions) with a severe loss in comprehension (*transcortical sensory aphasia*). In other cases, good comprehension and somewhat distorted production may be accompanied by an inability to repeat some simple phrase to an examiner (*conduction aphasia*).

One last specific syndrome is very rare: *isolation of the speech area*. Patients in this situation cannot converse with someone nor understand them, yet are capable of repeating, completing sentences, producing automatic sequences, and of correcting faulty grammar in a phrase that is repeated! Meaningful comprehension and production are impossible. In this rare condition, the speech areas are sufficiently intact, but they are isolated from other areas of the brain that produce the thoughts worth speaking. Thus, as shown in Figure 2.1, the commands of the examiner can be processed as sounds and word units, but meaning cannot be abstracted. The patient's own thoughts cannot be encoded into speech. One such patient was quite capable of learning new commercial jingles and songs, but not of holding a conversation.[6]

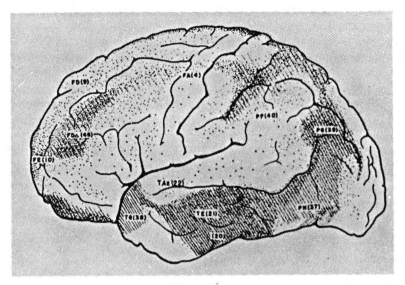

FIGURE 2.1. In this case, the speech areas of the left hemisphere have been totally isolated, yet left intact. See the text for a discussion of the syndrome. Reprinted by permission from Geschwind, Quadfasel & Segarra (1968).

There is also a syndrome of *global aphasia,* in which there is so much damage that virtually no language skills remain. The various combination of symptoms are summarized in Table 2.1 and many excellent summaries can be found with more detail.[7] Attempts to explain how the various aphasias come about range considerably, depending on the extent to which the author of the theory subscribes to a localizationist or a holistic view. For example, one localizationist approach is described by Norman Geschwind, who accounts for many syndromes by tracing the effects of disconnecting one area from another, such as in the isolation syndrome.[8] Others with a more holistic approach prefer to localize not whole speech functions, such as meaning or grammar, but rather more primitive neuropsychological functions, considering speech to be a complex product of such functions.[9] In any case, there is no question when it comes to brain lateralization. It is generally the *left* hemisphere that is under discussion. Whatever the basic functions are that subserve language, they are represented to a much greater extent in the left hemisphere. Table 2.2 provides some figures on this asymmetry. Damage to

23

TABLE 2.1. Symptoms of main types of aphasia.
The retention of an ability is indicated by +, an impairment by −, and an asterisk indicates a difficulty involving substitution of words.

	COMPREHENSION	*PRODUCTION*	*REPETITION*
Broca's	+	−	−
Wernicke's	−	*	−
Conduction	+	*	−
Transcortical motor	+	−	+
Transcortical sensory	−	*	+
Isolation	−	−	+
Global	−	−	−

different areas within the left hemisphere can lead to different symptoms. This can be seen in composite pictures of the damage leading to the various syndromes. Despite variation produced by individual differences, the clearest separation is between the Broca and Wernicke syndromes (see Figure 2.2).

TABLE 2.2. Incidence of aphasia after surgery on the left versus right hemisphere in patients without brain injury before two years of age (from Penfield & Roberts, 1959).

	SIDE OF SURGERY			
	LEFT		*RIGHT*	
	Total	*Incidence of aphasia*	Total	*Incidence of aphasia*
Right-handed	157	115	196	1
Left-handed	18	13	15	1
Total	175	128	211	2

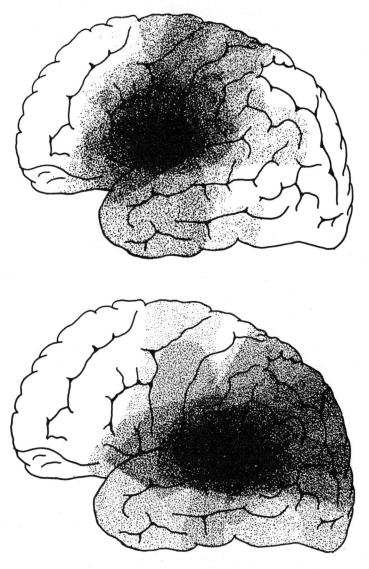

FIGURE 2.2. Kertesz, Lesk & McCabe (1977) have constructed composite pictures of the lesions producing various aphasias. We see here composite brain scans indicating the site of damage in 14 Broca's aphasics (top figure) and 13 Wernicke's aphasics (bottom figure). Reprinted by permission.

Tests for language dominance. When a patient must undergo brain surgery to remove a tumor or the focus of excessive epileptic discharge, it is crucial to determine where in the brain that person's language functions are represented. The locations of speech areas in the brain are not obvious before the operation for two reasons. First, everyone's brain is different in size and shape, just as faces are all different despite overall commonalities. As well, the pattern of representation of functions may be unique to some extent for each individual. In patients being prepared for brain surgery, the variability is much greater because their brains may have been affected by the disease process.

Two techniques have been developed to localize the speech centers, so the surgeon can be very careful to disturb these areas as little as possible. The first technique, developed by Juhn Wada in 1960, involves injecting a barbituate into the artery feeding one side of the brain. The drug, sodium amytal, temporarily paralyses the side injected. During the two or three minutes that the side is paralyzed, the patient is tested for speech. If the left side receives the injection, the typical response is a right-sided paralysis and a global or near global aphasia. As the drug is washed out of the brain's blood supply, full functions return. In this way, there can be no doubt about the probable effects of surgically induced damage to the side tested. This procedure is called the *Wada test*.

Another way of probing the brain for language representation involves electrically stimulating specific places on the cortex and charting the results. This is done, of course, in the operating room while the patient's brain is exposed. Only a local anesthetic need be used, so the patient is fully conscious and can report his thoughts and experiences. Electrical stimulation of a wide area in the left hemisphere interferes with speech, while in the right hemisphere, only stimulation in motor and some sensory areas interferes with speech. This latter interference is probably not a disruption of the conceptual processes in speech, but rather of motor processes. Right hemisphere stimulation in the temporal lobe (homologous to speech areas in the left hemisphere) produces hallucinations and perceptual illusions without speech interference.[10]

From the clinical literature on aphasia, it is clear that language functioning is more closely tied to the integrity of the left hemisphere than of the right. The variety of possible aphasic symptoms correlates to some extent with the location of the damage. Frontal (or *anterior*) lesions produce difficulties in planning and organizing the movements necessary for speech, lesions in the rear (or *posterior*) portions are more likely to produce semantic difficulties. Despite the outline of types of aphasia, many patients do not demonstrate the symptoms of any single type of aphasia, but are likely to show signs of various syndromes. This may be due to the brain damage not being restricted to a discrete area, or to our naive classification of disorders. The classification system has, however, proved useful for both descriptive and research purposes.

Finally, one question often asked is whether aphasia affects intelligence. To my mind, the answer depends on the questioner's assumptions about the concept of intelligence. Certainly most measures of intelligence are biased towards verbal skills. However, one gets the feeling with many aphasics, especially of the Broca type, that there is a great deal of thinking that is blocked because of the language deficit. But rather than surmise about the intellectual level of the aphasic, it is more profitable to consider the syndrome in detail and examine the specific skills still available to the individual.

Apraxia

A patient may have normal strength and coordination in his hands and normal comprehension, and yet be unable to carry out the purposeful movements needed to manipulate everyday items appropriately, such as lighting a candle. The patient may attempt to strike the match backwards, or strike the candle on the box and light the match with the candle. Or else the patient, again with strength and knowledge of what is required, may not be able to wave goodbye or make a sign of the cross.

This disorder is called *apraxia*. Sometimes the impossible action involves conventional signs, as in the latter examples, and sometimes real objects. The interesting aspect from our point of view is that often left hemisphere damage is critical for these disorders. The planning of movement seems to depend on left hemisphere integrity. This has been tested explicitly by comparing the speed and skill of hand and arm movements in patients with left- versus right-sided damage. Naturally damage to either side of the brain produced some weakness in the hand opposite the side of damage. But only the left brain-damaged group showed a decrease in skill in both hands.[11] Similarly, Doreen Kimura[12] has found that left brain-damaged patients, whether aphasic or not, have a great deal more difficulty learning a very simple series of motor tasks, as shown in Figure 2.3. The greatest difficulty the left-damaged group had was with *perseverative* errors, where a movement is inappropriately repeated (sometimes involuntarily). As well, the left-damaged group performed a number of unrelated, amorphous movements. The right-damaged group had no errors of these types at all. Kimura suggests, then, that the special function of the left hemisphere is the planning of movements. Since speech requires a great deal of fine coordination (several hundred muscular events every second), she suggests that this is why language is generally left-lateralized.

Right-Sided Damage and Apraxia. *Constructional apraxia,* a deficit in the ability to draw a copy from a model, can be due to either

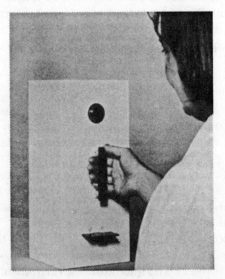

FIGURE 2.3. Left hemisphere damaged patients could not master the sequenced motor patterns needed for this task: pushing a button, pulling a handle, and depressing a lever. From Kimura (1977). Reprinted by permission.

left- or right-sided damage, both causing a difficulty in coordinating the visual image with the motor movements for drawing. The right damage produces a problem at the visual-spatial end of the task, the left damage at the motor-organization end.[13]

Another type of apraxia, sometimes considered to be an extreme form of the right-sided constructional disorder, is *dressing apraxia*. In this oddly specialized deficit, the patient cannot orient and place his clothing appropriately with respect to his body.

> He manipulates the clothes incoherently, turning and reversing them and handling them haphazardly. If by accident, he successfully accomplishes the task of laying out the clothes properly, prior to putting them on, he is unable to organize the gestures necessary to establish the appropriate relationship between his clothes and his body. The semiautomatic motor capacity for dressing oneself is lost. In most cases clothes may eventually be put on properly, after a series of fruitless attempts and after long reflection. Even in these cases, however, the patient is unable to tie a necktie or shoelaces.[14]

Keep in mind that this same patient does not seem clumsy or disoriented otherwise. Presumably there is some intellectual impairment leading to these symptoms, but the obvious manifestation is in this isolated but common behavior. There are other disorders that intrude into everyday living in surprisingly specific ways. For example, in facial agnosia, as mentioned before, the patient no longer recognizes faces, even his own.

The site of brain damage associated with constructional and dressing apraxia is the posterior region of the right side (in the area of the junction of the parietal, occipital and temporal lobes). The involvement of this area in visual and spatial processing accounts for the disorders, but not for their specificity. It may be that the tasks that are disturbed involve actions that are more intricate and complex than we usually imagine, since we take them for granted. It is only in their breakdown that we realize how complicated they really are. If this is the case, then these disturbed behaviors are isolated because they are indeed more difficult than others in some, as yet unarticulated, way. By comparison, posterior left hemisphere lesions (in the parietal-temporal area) underlie the non-constructional apraxias mentioned at the beginning of this section, presumably by disturbing the planning and sequencing skills of the individual.

From the clinical literature, we see that the importance of the parietal-temporal regions in completing planned activity is underscored. Damage to this area can substantially incapacitate a person's ability to function in everyday activities, although the cause of the problem differs for left- versus right-sided damage.

We should note that, although the various syndromes are described as separate entities, considerable controversy exists as to whether some types are simply weaker or stronger forms of others, or combinations of others.[15] In this summary, we have not done justice at all to the complexity of the problem of apraxia and the near-heroic efforts some researchers have shown in trying to make sense of this syndrome. Of course, in order to prove a differentiation between two syndromes, one must find for each type individuals who have one but not the other disturbance. Double dissociation is difficult to find with many apraxic symptoms, since often the patient has multiple difficulties. For example, various forms of apraxia are usually confounded with each other and with some aphasic symptoms as well.

Agnosia

In 1881, H. Munk described cases of what he called *psychic blindness* in a dog, produced by specific lesions in the visual cortex. The dog could walk freely around a room, jumping over obstacles without bumping into objects. However, it could not comprehend the meaning of the objects. For example, although hungry and thirsty, it ignored food and water. It did not retreat from threats, did not recognize its master, nor react to the presence of other dogs. It reacted like a dog newly brought into the world. In this case, the dog recovered and acted normally after a few weeks.

Visual Agnosias.   In people, *agnosia* refers to a loss of knowledge in a patient with intact sense perception. The visual agnosias are the best documented, although even they are rare in pure form. In *visual object agnosia*, for example, there is no loss of sight, but when presented with an object, a patient cannot name it or describe its usage verbally or with gestures, and yet can describe its shape and outline. Once allowed to touch, smell, or listen to the object (assuming it has a characteristic feel, odor or sound), the patient immediately recognizes it. For example, one patient called a bicycle, "a pole with two wheels, one in front, one in back" and a hat, a "little pot."[16] The loss is not always complete, since placing the object within its usual context often prompts recognition, just as some aspect of the object may give enough of a clue to permit a good guess. Still, the patient recognizes his identification as a guess and not as true recognition.

The damage causing this disorder is hard to specify because of the rarity of the syndrome. Of the few cases that have been well documented, there generally is bilateral damage, with the left occipital area critically involved. This contrasts with facial agnosia, described at the beginning of this chapter, in which bilateral damage is implicated, with an emphasis on the right-sided lesion.

Auditory Agnosia.   As we have seen, the underlying cause of the visual agnosias is not so clearly a lateralized lesion. The case is more clearly one of cerebral asymmetry with the auditory agnosias. For example, the loss of ability to recognize sounds, both everyday noises and musical pitch, can be present without aphasia. This loss is associated with damage to only the right hemisphere in regions analogous to those needed for word meaning in the left hemisphere.[17]

On the other hand, a patient with *pure word deafness* must have left hemisphere damage. Such a person can read, write and talk but cannot comprehend. Although the brain damage associated with the disorder is usually bilateral, several cases of unilateral lesions have been reported. In these cases, the damage must include the fibers feeding the left primary auditory area and the callosal connections from the right auditory area. Thus the patient can hear (via the right hemisphere), but this information cannot get directly to the language areas.[18] This syndrome is very rare since neither Broca's area or Wernicke's area may be involved (otherwise aphasia would ensue), and yet the auditory cortex must be damaged or isolated. Despite its rareness, this syndrome is instructive in clarifying the functional roles of the various areas in the left hemisphere.

Musical skills form a mixed set, some of which require left-hemisphere integrity, and some of which require right hemisphere functioning. Inasmuch as music is analogous to language without involving speech directly, it has been considered a right hemisphere skill. For example, Brenda Milner compared the musical skills of patients before and after surgical removal of a temporal lobe. All patients were known to be left-dominant for language. She presented a selection from the standard Seashore Measures of Musical Talents and found no drop in scores for the patients undergoing left temporal lobe removal. The right lobe patients dropped significantly on the tests of time duration, loudness, timbre, and tonal memory.[19] Similarly, when the right hemisphere is incapacitated temporarily by the Wada test, singing is grossly disturbed. Although rhythmic elements are maintained, the melody is reduced to monotones and random meandering.[20]

Case studies of musicians who sustain brain damage indicate, however, that when music is a highly developed skill, a right hemisphere predominance is not always complete. For example, Maurice Ravel suffered aphasia at the peak of his career. It was a Wernicke's aphasia, impairing oral and written language without a noticeable intellectual weakening, but complicated by an apraxia. The left hemisphere damage (presumed because of the aphasia) did not, however, affect Ravel's musical thinking.

> Recognition of tunes played before our musician is generally good and prompt. He recognizes immediately most of the works he knew, and anyway he recognizes perfectly his own works . . . he is able to evaluate exactly rhythm and style . . . He immediately notices the lightest mistake in the playing: several parts of the "Tombeau de Couperin" were first correctly played, and then with minor errors (either as to notes or rhythm). He immediately protested and demanded a perfect accuracy . . . my piano—because of the dampness of the winter—had become somewhat out of tune. The patient noticed it and demonstrated the dissonance . . .[21]

Unfortunately, in dramatic contrast to this retained clarity of musical thought, recognition of notes and musical dictation were highly impaired. Also, piano playing became too difficult and the writing down of notes either by himself or by dictation was well-nigh impossible. Thus, the productive part of his musical life was arrested by the aphasia.

There are other cases, however, where aphasia does not stop productive musical activities. The Russian composer, V. G. Shebalin, was slowed down, but managed to continue composing and teaching after suffering Wernicke's aphasia. A conductor, despite a gross Wernicke's aphasia, continued to lead his orchestra as did a professional pianist.[22] Musical skills, then, are dissociated from language skills, despite their highly structured, even "grammatical" qualities.[23] Whether or not a musical career will be disrupted by left-hemisphere damage depends both on the extent of the damage and the demands of the career (e.g., whether or not writing is required).

The Hemi-Spatial Neglect Syndrome

Some patients, such as the third case described on page one, show a loss not of specific skills or knowledge, but of attention to the left side of their personal space. Such patients may disavow their own left arm, or ignore some object to their left, although their vision is actually unimpaired. Rather, they chose not to attend to that side, although they will if the item on the left is brought to their attention. Thus, artists with the neglect syndrome leave unfinished the left side of the picture; when asked to draw a clock, the patient will try to cram all 12 hour markings into the right side of the circle; hungry patients may ignore the food on the left side of the plate.

Hemi-spatial neglect is very rarely seen in patients with left-sided damage, although this may be because it is not recognized as such: the language disturbance may overshadow any neglect symptoms.

Sorting Out Aphasias, Apraxias, and Agnosias

Agnosias, apraxias, and aphasias are examined through clinical case studies, and therefore conclusions are based on damaged or malfunctioning brains. Separating syndromes is a monumental task, but it is highly useful when successful. One of the reasons unambiguous results are not always found is that most tasks permit more than one strategy for solution, and these strategies may depend on different brain sites.[24] In order to detect such a complexity, we would have to find a task that definitely allows only one strategy (a very difficult undertaking since the concept of "strategy" itself may be interpreted at many levels), or find patients with lesions in all relevant sites. Otherwise, conflicting results will be found. Unfortunately, it is entirely possible that the strategies that patients have may depend in large measure on the strategies they developed before the trauma, that is, in individual differences existing before brain damage. Presumably, there are commonalities among all human minds, but there clearly are also differences. If these differences determine how neuropsychological tasks are attempted, the results are bound to become more variable (see Part IV for a more detailed discussion of individual differences).

Loss of all skill in a simple task from a unilateral lesion implies that no other region—especially the homologous one on the other side—can substitute at all. This is quite different from saying that one side is superior in the skill. For example, next to no substitution is possible with language production. It is very difficult for any other brain area to take over this function. However, this restriction is not so great in facial recognition. Different strategies are available to the patient for this task. In the next few chapters, we will discuss experimental work that clearly demonstrates a right hemisphere superiority in facial recognition. Yet for a complete loss of this ability, the damage must almost always be bilateral.

Recovery of Function
After Brain Damage

After brain damage has occurred, the patient may lose some functions. Almost always, however, he experiences some recovery as long as he survives the original trauma. How does such recovery occur? Two logical possibilities exist: Either the damaged area itself recovers to some degree or the function is served by different areas. As we will see, this issue is crucial to the question of localization of function.

Physiological Recovery of Damaged Tissue. When a brain region experiences some trauma, neurons are damaged and there is swelling in the region. With time, providing there is the normal recovery pattern, the swelling will reduce, allowing for the resumption of near normal activity by the undamaged cells in the area. For this reason alone, we expect some recovery.

Another consequence of brain trauma is that damaged but alive neurons regenerate connections. This "sprouting" may compensate for some of the lost connections. Also, there is some evidence that a change in biochemical sensitivity occurs after neuron damage, allowing a more sensitive response by the malfunctioning cells.[25]

Reorganization.

Regeneration of damaged tissue can account for only a fraction of the recovery of function, although no one yet knows the extent possible solely through these means. Much more dramatic is the reorganization of the function within the brain.

An example is provided by a recent experiment done on monkeys. After a destruction of part of one frontal lobe, monkeys seem to neglect the side opposite to the damage. They retreat from a threatening stimulus from either side, but if threatened on both sides simultaneously, they react only to the one on the same side as the lesion. Recovery from this unilateral neglect is fairly swift, often within two to three weeks. Is attention to the previously neglected side now mediated by some other area in the damaged hemisphere, by some recovery in the damaged area itself, or by the other side of the brain? The investigators surmised that it was the other hemisphere that could now mediate attention to both sides. They showed this by cutting the corpus callosum that connects the two sides. The one-sided deficit was restored, indicating that indeed the function had been mediated by the healthy side.[26]

Similarly, when people lose some skill through brain damage, they somehow mobilize the remaining resources to compensate as best they can. Some functions recover better than others. For example, Henri Hécaen reports that patients who have had the left occipital lobe removed recover the ability to read almost totally. However, in cases where more than the occipital lobe was lost, recovery was not good.[27] Thus, the initial loss of reading due to an occipital lobectomy can be compensated for by the regions immediately surrounding that area. However, if this surrounding area is also damaged, recovery is poor. Similarly, in some kinds of aphasia, the prognosis is good, in others it is poor.

How does a brain area that was not responsible for a function later become adequate for it? Luria describes it this way.[28] Each behavioral function depends on primary and secondary regions in the brain. One behavioral function, such as walking, speaking, or remembering faces, may depend on a number of cerebral functions localized in specific regions. These regions each interact with each other in various ways. When brain damage occurs, the balance is disrupted. The hampered cerebral function may be absolutely basic to the behavioral function, in which case recovery will be minimal. But there may be some way to compensate, some alternate strategy that allows the behavioral function to be retrieved. Such reorganization may end up including almost any of the cerebral cortex.[29]

This sounds like a difficulty for the localizationist position, since many (maybe most) functions can be compensated for. However, we still have to accept that some regions are more primary for certain functions than others. It is just that redundancies exist. Also, we should keep in mind that the recovery is seldom literal: Often the behavioral function is reachieved by a change in strategy. The patient changes the task to suit his remaining abilities.

There are two main spots in the brain to look for a regained ability: areas adjacent to the damage (as in Hécaen's example above), and the homologous area in the opposite hemisphere (as with the monkey example). Many functions are lost only when the damage is bilateral, indicating that the opposite hemisphere often compensates. The most dramatic example is when patients do recover some use of language after aphasia. There can be no doubt where the mediation is for recovered speech when the entire left hemisphere is removed.[30] In cases of aphasia suffered through strokes or accidents, the source of recovery is less certain, although it is mediated at least occasionally by the previously nondominant right hemisphere.[31]

How can the right hemisphere, incapable of speech just before the injury, develop the ability? We presume that the loss of the entire left hemisphere has two effects: most obviously a loss of left hemisphere functions, but also a removal of inhibition of the right hemisphere for those functions.[32] When we say that the left hemisphere is *dominant* for speech, we mean just that—it dominates in the control of speech. Whether or not the right hemisphere will have the ability to compensate after the loss of the left is another issue.[33]

Language and the Right Hemisphere

We have characterized the right hemisphere as nonverbal until it is forced into language requirements by a loss of the left hemisphere. This implies that the right hemisphere is normally not involved in language use at all and is misleading inasmuch as language and communication are not simple, unitary functions. There is no doubt that the left hemisphere is dominant for the traditional "compartments" of language: sounds (phonology), grammar (syntax), and meaning (semantics). There are, however, some subtle language-related activities that do seem to involve the right hemisphere.

Intonation.　The intonation pattern in speech—the rises and drops in pitch and loudness—not only indicates emphasis and emotional tone, but also gives some grammatical cues. Although aphasics show a clear loss of grammatical skills, some such ability is preserved and can be mediated through the use of intonation. For example, although a Broca's aphasic seems to have lost intonation because his speech is so fragmented, a careful analysis indicates that the correct pattern is used (with obvious gaps) to specify a statement versus a question.[34]

Right hemisphere damaged patients present a very different profile. Their speech seems all right, since pronunciation and grammar are acceptable although there can be a flattening of intonation. However, their judgments of the emotional tone of sentences said by others is worse than that of aphasics, although they can understand the content satisfactorily.[35] For example, a woman who had a stroke in the right hemisphere in the region homologous to Broca's area on the other side, presented symptoms that were considerably disruptive although more subtle than those of an aphasic. The emotional inflection was gone from her voice. Her tone was flat and thus her speech was considerably less effective than usual. Since she was a schoolteacher, this was extremely disruptive. Since

she usually maintained classroom discipline through the affective quality of her speech, she found it impossible to adequately control her students. Her own children were also hard to discipline because they, too, could not detect when she was angry, upset, or really "meant

37

business." She was able to circumvent these difficulties at home by tacking a parenthetical statement, such as "God damn it, I mean it" or "I am angry and mean it," after a sentence, but it should be emphasized that even the parenthetical statement was voiced in a complete monotone without emotion, as were other profanities and expletives. The patient had also lost her ability to cry and laugh. While attending her father's funeral, she was totally unable to express emotion although inwardly she was sad and wanted to cry. When she finally "forced" herself to cry, her husband noted that it sounded stilted, unconvincing, and entirely different from her usual crying. The patient stated that her ability to experience emotion was not impaired, only its outward expression. She reported no difficulties perceiving other people's emotions through their use of speech intonations, facial expressions, or gestures.[36]

The right hemisphere basis for intonation has been exploited in therapy. Martin Albert, Robert Sparks, and Nancy Helm have developed a program called Melodic Intonation Therapy, whereby aphasics are taught phrases in song, since singing is often preserved in aphasia while voluntary sentence construction is not. Gradually, the melodic part of the sequence is deemphasized, until the patient has at his command the phrase alone. If the patient has difficulty, he reverts temporarily to an intoned response. By using the right hemisphere intonation skills, the new strategy can be used to accommodate some speech. For example,

> a 67-year old man had been unable to produce language for 18 months following a stroke. His comprehension was good, but his output was limited to meaningless grunts. During the course of his illness, he had received three months of language therapy with no success. Two days after beginning melodic intonation therapy he produced a few words. In two weeks he had a usable verbal output of approximately 100 words. After 1½ months he carried on short, meaningful conversations, many of which he spontaneously initiated.[37]

Not all aphasics respond so positively to melodic intonation therapy. Just for whom it is appropriate and how it works is still being debated. However, the developers of the therapy suggest that it will be most effective with patients who have good comprehension but inadequate production; that is, the language blockage must be at the output end. Presumably the change in strategy (using melody to prompt articulation) is successful because it is mediated by the undamaged right hemisphere, which is normally incapable of voluntary speech production. The alternate strategy exploited by this therapy may lift the inhibition.

     Speech Acts. A speech act refers to a function of language, which may or may not be apparent from the surface meaning of the utterance. For example, in order to receive the salt shaker at the dinner table, one can request it in a number of ways (varying in politeness, among other things): "Please pass the salt", "Do you have any salt?", "Can anyone see the salt?", or "This soup needs more salt!" Some requests are phrased as questions, some as statements, some as commands, and some as offhand comments. Still, they are all requests. The conversational effect that a sentence has, called its *illocutionary force*, depends on context and the culture, as well as grammar.[38] Left hemisphere damaged patients with aphasia can interpret the illocutionary force required by a situation, although they may not be able to express it fluently. Similarly, when presented with a story, aphasics may choose to interpret a sentence directly or indirectly. For example, the patient can be given the context: "A student has an interview with his professor. The window is wide open. The student says to the professor, 'I have a very bad cold.' " The patient is given the option of interpreting the student's utterance as (1) a request, (2) a complaint, (3) a contradiction, or (4) a command. In contrast with aphasics, right hemisphere damaged patients tend to choose the literal interpretation (number 2).[39] They seem to lack the ability to integrate subtle clues into a single concept, to make global sense of the situation. This tendency towards literalness is demonstrated even more dramatically in their treatment of metaphor and humor, discussed next.

     Metaphor and Humor. Much of language is figurative, with the intended meaning an extension of the literal meaning of the words used. Many of these extensions deal with analogies of experiences from the various senses (I *see* what you mean; a *hard* heart; a *loud* tie; *rough* times; a movie that *stinks*). The meaningful application of a word referring to one of the senses in another context is not self-evident. It can vary across languages and children take years to develop a sense of metaphor.[40] Appreciation of metaphor also varies among aphasics, right brain-damaged patients, and normals.

Ellen Winner and Howard Gardner presented a series of sentences to subjects and asked which of four response pictures best corresponded to the sentence.[41] For example, for the sentence "A heavy heart can really make a difference," the subject could choose an appropriate metaphoric picture (a person crying), a literal rendition (a person staggering under the weight of a large red heart), a picture emphasizing the adjective (a 500 lb. weight), or one representing the noun (a red heart). Normals gave about five times as many metaphorical responses as literal responses, aphasics over three times as many, while right hemisphere patients responded with equal frequency to the metaphorical and literal choices. Interestingly, the aphasics emphatically rejected the literal depictions, often laughing at the absurdities, while right hemisphere patients seemed indifferent.

A similar situation is found with the appreciation of humor. Aphasics enjoy cartoons in the same way as normals, while right hemisphere patients often miss the point unless it is given in a caption.[42] When given a set of endings for a joke, these patients prefer non sequiturs that provide surprise, which is appropriate, but lack the tie-in to the context that is necessary.[43] Interestingly, this pattern is also demonstrated in young children, where they enjoy the incongruity of a non-sequitur in riddles, but do not see the requirement for the answer to make sense as well.[44] This lack in children is seen as an inability to see how the pieces of the riddle (the questions and the response) fit together. Presumably, a similar function is disrupted with right-sided brain damage.

Conceptual Disruption with Right Hemisphere Damage. Despite the linguistic nature of some of the tasks described above, aphasics perform more normally on them than do right hemisphere patients. When asked to retell a parable-like story they have just heard, aphasics naturally have difficulty, but can, nonetheless, make clear the main events, the motivations of the characters and give the moral of the story. Right hemisphere patients can relate the major events, but have difficulty inferring the motivations and feelings of the characters. They also have great difficulty extracting an appropriate moral from the story.[45]

Right brain damaged subjects also have difficulty on "two-term series" problems with antonymic adjectives, such as this one: John is taller than Bill, who is shorter?[46] Although this could be solved purely verbally, the impairment shown by the patients implies that the usual strategy involves imagery at some level. Once again, "putting the scene together" is difficult for these patients.

Despite the clear involvement of the left hemisphere in language functions, the right side is necessary for normal communication in a broader sense. The usual standardized tests of linguistic ability focus on pronunciation and grammar. In these, the left hemisphere is clearly dominant. But the behavioral function of language is more complex than that, and for normal activity multiple cerebral functions are necessary. These studies on right hemisphere patients demonstrate the interdependence of the two hemispheres in normal functioning, as well as the inadequacy of the notion that one hemisphere can be completely dominant over the other in normal (complex) behavior.

Left Versus Right
Hemisphere Syndromes

Having covered considerable ground in this chapter, let us now try to summarize the clinical findings of symptoms associated with left- and right-hemisphere damage. To do so, of course, will involve simplification, but hopefully the subtleties ignored here will be adequately emphasized later.

The left hemisphere involvement in language skills is most obvious, with a variety of possible symptoms. A conceptual division groups the frontal areas with the planning and organization of speech and the posterior areas with semantic functions. These semantic functions include relational ideas. For example, Luria describes semantic aphasia as including a disturbance of calculation ability. The patient cannot figure out how the numbers relate in simple addition when the problem is written in a nonstandard way (see Figure 2.4). Similarly, he cannot solve relational requests such as, "How are you and your father's brother related?" or, "Put the cup on the block." The patient understands the items to be related, but cannot figure out the direction of the relation.[47]

The right hemisphere is especially involved in visual-spatial and melodic skills. Because these are less crucial to normal

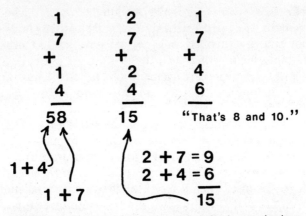

FIGURE 2.4. The patient with semantic aphasia can also lose the semantic structure of numbers, producing these results. These same patients can easily solve problems in the usual orientation.

functioning and perhaps also open to compensation, the degree of right hemisphere dominance appears to be less for these skills than the degree of left-hemisphere dominance for language. However, some subtle characteristics are disrupted more by right-sided brain damage than by left-sided damage: expression of emotion and feelings, inference of others' feelings and motivations, and a sense of humor. The right hemisphere, then, seems to be necessary for integrating information and making inferences from that synthesis, especially when dealing with visual or nonverbal material.

NOTES

1. Occasionally graphic symbols, such as a red cross or swastika, are also unrecognized, although well perceived (Benton, 1979).
2. Gardner (1974), Heilman & Valenstein (1979), Hećaen & Albert (1978), Segalowitz (1983).
3. This and the following example are reported in Goodglass (1976).
4. Their difficulty may be due to not knowing what to do with the omitted words as much as difficulties in saying them. See Zurif & Caramazza (1976).

5. Luria (1966a).
6. Geschwind, Quadfasel & Segarra (1968). Whitaker (1976) presents a more detailed linguistic analysis of the remaining skills of another isolation case.
7. Goodglass & Kaplan (1972), Benson (1979), Dingwall & Whitaker (1974), Hécaen & Albert (1978), Luria (1966a), Geschwind (1972), Goodglass & Geschwind (1976), Kertesz (1979).
8. Geschwind (1965, 1972).
9. Luria (1966a, b), Lenneberg (1975).
10. Penfield & Roberts (1959), Ojemann & Whitaker (1978).
11. Wyke (1971).
12. Kimura & Archibald (1974), Kimura (1977).
13. Hécaen & Albert (1978).
14. Hécaen & Albert (1978, p. 106).
15. Hécaen & Albert (1978, chapter 3); Geschwind (1965).
16. Hécaen & Albert (1978, p. 195); see also Rubens (1979) for a summary of the agnosias.
17. Spreen, Benton & Fincham (1965).
18. See Albert & Baer (1974), Rubens (1979) or Hécaen & Albert (1978) for more details.
19. Milner (1962).
20. Bogen & Gordon (1971) discuss six cases; Mosidze (1976) presents another four.
21. See Alajouanine (1948), who also discusses aphasia in an artist and a writer. Several brief summaries of the effects of brain damage on artistic endeavors are given in Gardner (1974, Chapter 8).
22. Luria, Tsvetkova & Futer (1965); Gardner (1974, p. 338); Assal (1973).
23. Jackendoff (mimeo); Bernstein (1976).
24. See Hécaen & Albert (1978, p. 230–231) for an example of this problem in visual-spatial perception.
25. See Kolb & Whishaw (1980, Chapter 19) and Jacobson (1978) for more details.
26. Crowne, Yeo & Russell (1981).
27. As described in Hécaen & Albert (1978, p. 381).
28. Luria (1966a, b; 1970a).
29. Luria (1963).
30. Smith (1966), Dennis (1980).

31. Kinsbourne (1971).
32. Moscovitch (1977).
33. Several factors are at play here, the most crucial being the developmental history of the inhibition. When the inhibition is lacking from very early on, either because of a lack of connection between the hemispheres along which to mediate the suppression (agenesis of the corpus callosum) or because of early hemispherectomy, the right hemisphere is quite capable of developing language (Dennis & Whitaker, 1977; Netley, 1977).
34. Danly & Shapiro (1982), Danly, Cooper & Shapiro (in press), and as summarized in Foldi, Cicone & Gardner (in press).
35. Heilman, Scholes & Watson (1975).
36. Ross & Mesulam (1979).
37. Albert, Sparks & Helm (1973); see also Sparks, Helm & Albert (1974).
38. Searle (1969); Austin (1962).
39. Heeschen & Reisches (1979, cited in Foldi, Cicone & Gardner, 1983).
40. Cometa & Eson (1978), Malgady (1977).
41. Winner & Gardner (1977).
42. Gardner, Ling, Flamm & Silverman (1975).
43. Work by Michel & Gardner, described in Foldi, Cicone & Gardner (1983).
44. Shultz (1974), McGhee (1974).
45. Wapner, Hamby & Gardner (1981).
46. Caramazza, Gordon, Zurif & Deluca (1976). See also Gardner, Silverman, Wapner & Zurif (1978) for the relative appreciation of synonyms and antonyms in left and right hemisphere patients.
47. Luria (1966, 1969).

chapter three

Separating
the left brain
from the right brain

Let not thy left hand know
What thy right hand doest.
Matthew VI, 3

How many times have all of us felt as if we had two independent minds, each quite different, sometimes even contradictory—and not only when we are contemplating charity, as St. Matthew would have us do. In some individuals, however, the duality of purpose or of consciousness is not metaphorical at all, but concrete and demonstrable. Several decades ago, it was discovered that some forms of intractable epilepsy could be relieved by cutting the connections, called the *commissures*, between the cerebral hemispheres. By performing a *commissurotomy*, as the operation is called, the spreading activation of the seizure cannot cross to the other side. Often these split-brain patients seem so normal that the cerebral commissures that connect the two sides were facetiously deemed to have no function at all except to transmit epilepsy! Indeed, there was considerable doubt as to whether any symptoms ensue from commissurotomy at all.[1]

More recently, however, a series of laboratory case studies have shown that relatively subtle symptoms can be found in split-brain patients if they are looked for carefully. By separating the hemispheres, information received by only one hemisphere cannot cross to the other side. In ordinary life experiences, it is rare that information should be so selectively received, so that split-brain patients are relatively unaffected in their everyday life by the disconnection syndrome. Nevertheless, the disconnection can be demonstrated by taking advantage of sensory modalities that separate the input to the two hemispheres.

How to Tell
One Hemisphere Something
Without the Other Knowing

As a general rule, the left side of the brain controls the right side of the body, and vice versa. Like mose general rules, however, there are many exceptions, some of which will be discussed in the next chapter. Two of the senses that do follow the rule are touch and vision, so the disconnection apparent in split-brain patients can be studied using these modalities. For example, a patient is seated at a table with a barrier placed so that objects behind it can be felt with one hand, but cannot be seen (see Figure 3.1). When the subject feels, say, a comb with the right hand, he has no difficulty telling the experimenter what the object is. However, when the left hand is used, usually the subject can only hazard a guess. Presumably, this is because the information about the object is transmitted to the right hemisphere and is unavailable to the left, which is the one capable of responding verbally.[2] As we shall see, this does not mean that the subject does not understand what the object is, rather, only that a verbal response is impossible.

A visual task separates the input to each hemisphere in a way similar to the tactual one. Because of the way the visual system is connected, the left half of the visual field is projected to the right side of the brain and the right visual field to the left side. This division is for *both* eyes (see Figure 3.2). Thus, if the word TOMBOY is presented so that the center of the subject's visual field is between the middle two letters, then the right hemisphere receives TOM and the left receives BOY. The normal person, of course, automatically integrates these two parts to form the whole word. A commissurotomy patient, however, cannot integrate them, and will claim verbally

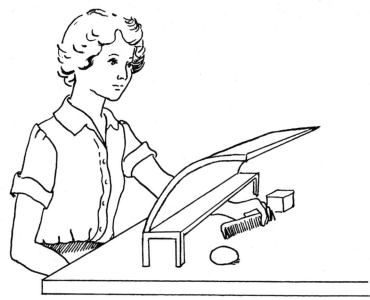

FIGURE 3.1. In this set-up, the split-brain patient must identify the object from touching it only. If language representation is limited to the left hemisphere, this cannot be done with the left hand.

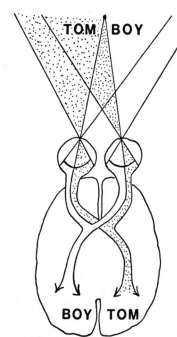

FIGURE 3.2. The human visual system is structured so that the field of vision to the left of fixation (for both eyes) projects to the right hemisphere and the right visual field to the left hemisphere. Thus, the split-brain patient in this figure would report (that is, the left hemisphere would report) that the word BOY was shown. The isolated right side would disagree if its opinion could be garnered. The normal subject, of course, integrates the two visual fields and so would see TOMBOY.

that only BOY was projected. If given a chance to feel with the left hand for objects whose names are flashed to the left visual field only (right hemisphere), the patient will usually pick out the correct object while claiming verbally all the while that no word was seen.

Such bizarre situations are easy enough to construct, if care is taken, and can tell us much about the isolated hemispheres. However, the split-brain subject does not feel that anything is bizarre. His verbal self (the left hemisphere) converses with the experimenter oblivious to the details of the right hemisphere's activities, and unaware of this ignorance. Usually this separation results in the conversing left hemisphere "faking it" as best it can. For example, in the experimental situations where care is taken to keep the left side ignorant of the input, the patient responds with a best guess, often a wild one, or a denial that any stimulus was presented. Simultaneously, however, the left hand may respond by picking out a correct object. Sometimes this dissociation, called the "alien hand" syndrome, is noticed by the patient and can be disturbing.

For example, Joseph Bogen describes a patient who complained of her "little sister" when trying to account for the behavior of her left hand.[3] The left hand even tries to correct the mistakes of the right hand on occasion. The feeling that the left side is foreign can extend to foot movements as well, creating difficulty in coordination. Generally, however, there is adaptation and the patient develops methods for transferring information from one hemisphere to the other (to be discussed later).

The Intellectual Strengths and Weaknesses of Each Separated Hemisphere

By extensive testing of the isolated hemispheres of split-brain patients, we know that the left hemisphere is vastly superior to the right on linguistic tasks in these patients. It responds accurately on all tests of word knowledge and usage, while the isolated right hemisphere does not. The right hemisphere is quite good in some patients at identifying word items from their pictures (sometimes even at a level of an 11-year-old), but the grammatical knowledge and phonetic skills are very poor (at most, like that of a 4- or 5-year-old).

Apparently verbs produce a greater difficulty for the isolated right hemisphere than do nouns, which could be due to greater abstractness or greater grammatical complexity.[4]

Nonlinguistic tasks, however, do not give as many problems to the lone right hemisphere. For example, when a line with a particular slope is flashed to the isolated hemispheres for identification, it is the right hemisphere that is better at identifying the angle. Similarly, the right hemisphere shows superior skill for copying designs, such as three dimensional cubes or Greek crosses, or for matching visually presented designs to felt templates. The right hemisphere-left hand system also shows superiority on part-whole matching problems, for example where an arc must be matched to a circle of the same size.[5]

What underlies the differences in talents between the hemispheres? To simply label the skills as "verbal" versus "spatial" may give a fairly accurate summary of the left-versus right-sided talents, but does not help us understand the processing differences between the hemispheres. A popular attempt at doing this attributes different cognitive styles to the hemispheres. For example, in the task involving tactually finding a pattern that fits a blank in a visually presented design, split-brain subjects showed different strategies with each hand.

> When identifying patterns with their right hand, subjects tended to work slowly and to verbalize their reasoning, giving verbal labels to aspects of the pattern such as number, distance or angle. By contrast, when working with the left hand, subjects' performance was much more rapid, confident and silent. Performance with the right hand was in all cases slower than with the left hand by 25%.[6]

It appears that the right-hand/left-hemisphere system prefers a sequential, detailed strategy while the left hand-right hemisphere prefers a more global tactic for identification of the stimulus. This difference between the hemispheres in strategy has recently been supported by a study with normals using the visual paradigm. Phyllis Ross and Gerald Turkewitz presented faces for identification in either the left or right visual field. As illustrated in Figure 3.2, the stimulus is initially received by the opposite hemisphere. With normals, however, the information then transfers to the other side.

They found that some people show an advantage in the right visual field (left hemisphere) and others in the left visual field (right hemisphere), indicating that the lead given to the left hemisphere was preferred by some, and to the right by others. In a subsequent experiment, individuals with the left hemisphere advantage were more easily disrupted by an obscuring of details on the faces (such as eyebrows or nose), while the performance of the others was disrupted more when global changes were made (by inverting the faces).[7] It appears, then, that the left hemisphere is more sensitive to details and the right is more sensitive to overall design.

Contrasting with the cognitive style hypothesis is the approach used by Michael Gazzaniga and Joseph LeDoux, who stress the response requirements of the tasks. They claim that with visual-spatial tasks, the isolated left hemisphere performs as well or nearly as well as the isolated right hemisphere. When the task requires manipulation of objects, however, the right hemisphere superiority becomes striking. They reject the cognitive style hypothesis, since the left hemisphere appears *capable* of spatial reasoning. Rather, they claim there is a specialization in the right hemisphere for organized manipulation of objects. At the moment, their claim is rather controversial since they have yet to account for the hemisphere differences found in normals on spatial tasks (which will be discussed in Chapter 6).[8]

How to Fake It
With a Hemispheric Separation:
Adaptation in the Separated Brain

As was mentioned earlier, the split-brain patient behaves quite normally in the real world. Even in laboratory situations he or she converses with the experimenter, and rarely acknowledges the effects of the commissurotomy. We can ask the patient (i.e. the left hemisphere) to tell us what was flashed when we have made sure that only the right hemisphere knows, but the patient still often comes up with a fairly good guess. How could this be so? Some information may transfer directly because of incomplete cutting of the corpus callosum, or through other of the uncut, small commissures. Alternatively, some information may be transferring indirectly. This latter flow of information includes *cross-cueing.*

Cross-cueing. Whether split-brained or not, we all continually act on incomplete information, making best guesses about the world. We do it whether we are making conscious guesses about how a colleague or spouse is feeling at the moment, or whether making automatic, unconscious decisions about the slipperiness of the sidewalk we are walking on. Often we only realize that we acted on incomplete information when we fall flat on our face, figuratively or literally. Similarly, the isolated, non-informed hemisphere guesses continually on partial information and is usually correct. Sometimes, the other hemisphere is able to cue the responding one, to help out.

For example, while testing the language skills of the right hemisphere, Michael Gazzaniga and Steven Hillyard found that the supposedly mute side could reliably report digits (the numbers two to nine). Whether the numbers were flashed to the left or right visual field, the subject could read them out. However, the reaction time for the right visual field-left hemisphere system was under one second for all digits, while the left visual field response required over two seconds for a *2* and increased gradually until five seconds were required for an *8*. When forced to answer quickly, accuracy dropped to chance levels. The subject volunteered that he had developed a strategy involving cross-cueing: "What I do (meaning what the left hemisphere does) is to count up until I hit a number that 'sticks out'. Then I stop and tell you what it is."[9] The right hemisphere could read the number, but not report it. It could, however, transfer a feeling to the other side, as a cue.

With another patient, an adolescent boy, Gazzaniga and his colleagues asked that the action described by the word flashed to the right hemisphere be performed. When *kiss* was shown, the boy (i.e., his left hemisphere) immediately responded, "Hey, no way, no way. You've got to be kidding." Yet he could not say what it was that he objected to. When *kiss* was flashed to the left hemisphere, he said, "No way. I'm not going to kiss you guys." This time the speaking side knew both the feeling and the reason.

Cross-cueing can be more overt. One subject, when asked to identify a picture of Hitler, was caught trying to trace the letter *H* with her left hand on the back of her right hand to cue the speaking hemisphere. Another time, the subject could tell that the word *boxer* had been flashed to the right hemisphere when he found himself clenching and raising his fists in a boxing position. When restrained, he could not tell what the word was. Sometimes the cues are misread. In response to *rub*, the subject rubbed the back of his head (with the left hand, of course), but responded with a good, but incorrect, guess—*itch*.[10]

Adapting to a Split-Brain. After a commissurotomy, the patient has a great deal of recovering to do beyond that required by the brain surgery. Hopefully the epilepsy is reduced to controllable proportions, this factor alone requiring considerable (happy) changes in his life. However, the two hemispheres also must relearn how to cooperate. As discussed in the last chapter, there is considerable room for recovery of function in terms of reorganization, and this reorganization may take months as the patient learns to cope with his new condition.

For example, one patient, named P.S., showed a dramatic change over the five month period following his operation. On a task where each hemisphere received a different face to recognize, he responded in the first month with each hemisphere selecting the appropriate stimulus (no dominance by one side or the other), and gradually moved to the right hemisphere choice dominating the response.[11] This functional change, a change in dominance for facial recognition, reflects the dynamic nature of the plasticity of the brain when recovering from damage.

By the same token, we should be wary about generalizing the specifics of brain lateralization in commissurotomy patients too freely to normals. Remember that these patients, P.S. in particular, may have suffered early brain trauma, and may have experienced some reorganization of unknown proportions even before the operation to split the hemispheres.

This can be seen more clearly in cases of *agenesis* of the corpus callosum, where the great commissure never develops in the first place. In such patients, language skills are often represented in both hemispheres and other compensations in brain development may have occurred, so that evidence of the agenesis is difficult to come by.[12] In addition, these people have had a lifetime of developing cross-cueing strategies so that they need not be conscious of them anymore. However, there are limits to the reorganization possible. Once cross-cueing is carefully controlled for, integration of visual information, fine motor, and tactile information is not complete.[13]

Not all Split-Brains Are Alike. It is important to keep in mind that to some extent each person is neuropsychologically unique. There are individual differences in neurological structures and, of course, wide individual differences in psychological makeup. Not surprisingly, there is quite some range in how psychological functions are represented in the brain. For example, Gail Risse showed that one of the minor commissures not always cut in the commissurotomy operation, the anterior commissure, transmits different information in different patients, indicating a source of difficulty in generalizing across all patients. Patients differed considerably in how much visual, auditory, olfactory, and tactual information could cross hemispheres.[14]

Split-brain patients are especially unique for two additional reasons: (1) early damage may have induced reorganization of functions, and (2) the commissurotomy operation is tailored to suit the needs of the patient. Sometimes the entire corpus callosum is cut, sometimes only part is cut. Sometimes the anterior commissure, one of the other minor connecting fibres, is left, sometimes it is cut also. This variability can be useful in addressing other questions. For example, Gazzaniga and LeDoux discuss the effects of sectioning only the part of the corpus callosum that joins the frontal lobes. In this patient, visual information could transfer from one hemisphere to the other (in the posterior portion of the brain). Interestingly, though, when the patient mentally constructed a visual image of an object felt by the right hand only, he could not pick it out with his left hand. When a picture of it was flashed to the left hemisphere, he had no problem picking it out. Thus, the visual experience crossed, but not the self-generated visual image, indicating that imaging involves more (or different) processes than the visual perceptual experience.[15]

Two Minds in One (Split-) Brain?

At the beginning of this chapter, we considered the existence of two minds in the same brain. There is now strong evidence that this can be taken quite literally in the case of commissurotomy subjects. For example, in a study with a commissurotomized monkey, one hemisphere had the temporal lobe removed to produce a distinct syndrome, one symptom of which is tameness with humans. When only the intact hemisphere could see, the monkey showed the usual reactions to humans—intense fear. When only the side with the temporal lobectomy could see, the monkey was docile with humans.[16] This is literally a "split personality". Whether something akin to this occurs with normal people who possess intact brains will be discussed below.

Human split-brain patients have often given evidence of possessing two somewhat differing minds. This is not the same as seeing both sides of an argument, which often happens to all of us. Rather, it involves being quite certain of two incompatible things at the same time. For example, the patient P.S. stated (i.e. his left hemisphere stated) that he wanted to be a draftsman when he grows up, yet his right hemisphere spelled out *automobile race* when asked what job it would pick. On another task, he was asked to indicate how much he liked or disliked a series of items that were flashed only to the left or to the right hemisphere. At the height of the Watergate scandal, the widest divergence between the two hemispheres on a like-dislike scale was the item *Nixon*—the right hemisphere expressed "dislike" while the left expressed "like."[17] Such dramatic differences in relatively subtle judgments are available because P.S's right hemisphere is quite verbally competent. Usually this is not the case in split brain patients. Rather, a more subtle dissociation between two parts of every personality, the verbal self and the emotional, nonverbal self can be seen.

For example, commissurotomy patients are less likely to talk about their feelings, as if they are not as available for discussion. Occasionally, there is direct conflict. Joseph Bogen reports that one patient's physiotherapist reported, "You should have seen Rocky yesterday—one hand was buttoning up his shirt and the other hand was coming right behind it undoing the buttons!"[18] Such working at cross-purposes can produce considerable consternation, where the left hand, as mentioned before, feels alien or foreign. Surely this is evidence of two (at least somewhat) separate minds in the same body!

The Split-Brain As a Model For Normal Brains

Is any of this relevant for normal brains? Are we all, in some manner, to some extent, split-brained? Certainly we all acknowledge the feeling of "being of two minds," although this is a euphemism for not being able to make up one's (single) mind. Are there times, however, when our intact brains act as if there were disconnections? Certainly this is commonplace in the most general sense, whenever we find that the word for some thought, feeling, or idea is unavailable. Consider the situation where we verbalize one desire and feel another. This is the basis for psychotherapy, in which the various parts of a patient conflict in their needs and the patient cannot keep in charge, often because he (i.e. his verbal self) does not understand or admit the needs of the nonverbal parts of his personality. This speculative issue will be discussed at more length in Chapter 14.

This idea can be used here to introduce Gazzaniga and LeDoux's notion of the *sociology of the mind*: that the human mind is made up of several parts—a verbal self, an emotional self, a motor-action self, etc.—and these parts can be separated on physiological as well as psychological or philosophical grounds. When the split-brain patient laughs at a picture presented to the right hemisphere and cannot say why he laughed, we know he isn't lying or hiding something but rather that his left (speaking) hemisphere didn't see the picture. Is it possible that when you or I make a "Freudian slip," we often do not know why for the same reason? Disconnections in the noncommissurotomized person need not only reflect left-right blockages. *Functional disconnections*, if they occur, may be temporary miscommunications for whatever reason.

Evidence for Functional Disconnections. There is plentiful evidence that parts of the central nervous system can act as if they have been physically disconnected. The most dramatic cases involve hysterical paralysis, in which the patient is partly paralyzed although there is no damage to the nervous system. Often, with psychological help, the blockage disappears. Hypnosis presents another convincing case where, upon an arbitrary suggestion, the subject can suppress certain sensory information. Functional disconnections, then, should not seem too strange for the normal (noncommissurotomized) subject to experience given the appropriate circumstances.

Can and does functional *hemispheric* disconnection occur, though? A complete functional disconnection would, of course, mimic the split-brain syndrome. This has never been reported in a noncommissurotomized patient and is highly unlikely to occur.

However, it is not odd to think of each hemisphere as functioning somewhat separately from the other—that is, that each side works as a unit within itself as well as the two sides working as a unit together. For example, we have many experiences where skills that are learned by one side of the body do not transfer to the other side. The fine skill of throwing a ball, writing, or playing a musical instrument does not transfer across hands automatically. R.E. Myers demonstrated how this coordination within a hemisphere is greater than coordination across hemispheres. He compared how well cats could learn two opposite responses in two different conditions: one where each hemisphere received opposite instructions, the other where the same hemisphere received the conflicting training. Thus, in the first condition, he taught one hemisphere to choose one symbol and to ignore another, and the other hemisphere the opposite responses. Naturally there was conflict since the information would transfer across the corpus callosum. However, the degree of conflict increased considerably in the second condition when he tried to teach one hemisphere both patterns.[19] This relative weakness of the *inter*hemispheric connections compared with the *intra*hemispheric connections has been shown repeatedly in animal studies.[20]

To generalize about humans in everyday activity, could it be that one hemisphere seems to "take charge," ignoring or even suppressing the activity of the other? If so, this would be quite analogous to a split-brain patient laughing at something shown only to the right hemisphere, without being able to describe the cause of the outburst. One way this might occur is by one hemisphere becoming more activated, thereby inhibiting the other's control on the subject's behavior. For example, Robert Ley recently reported a series of studies in which he prompted subjects to activate one hemisphere more than the other by having them remember a list of either highly emotion-laden words (e.g. rape, cancer) or emotionally neutral words. Before and after hearing the word list, each subject was given a test of cerebral dominance for speech (the dichotic listening task, which is described in the next chapter). The group with highly emotional words showed a shift towards right hemisphere control compared to the other group. Thus, with the relatively innocuous task of remembering a list of words in a laboratory, a differential change in hemisphere dominance could be produced.[21] We can expect that relative dominance (i.e. control over behavior) is constantly shifting in normal behavior, perhaps occasionally with two separate areas acting simultaneously and not interacting to any great extent.

Split-Brains Versus Normals: Pros and Cons

How much should we make of the split-brain literature? Does the work on right hemisphere language mean that in normals the non-speech hemisphere comprehends English at a 12-year-old's level? Does the finding that the right hand in the commissurotomy patient is remarkably inept at copying or drawing mean that in normals the left hemisphere is totally unartistic? In this summary, we will address the main arguments brought forward on each side of the debate.

   Cons.   Normals do not have split brains, therefore no direct application of split-brain results can be made. Attempts to dichotomize about left- and right-sided skills with normals is an example of such faulty thinking. This is precisely what has happened in the popular press, where the left hemisphere is characterized as linguistic, mathematical, scientific and logical while the right is characterized as responsible for music, art and dance appreciation, perception, sculpture, and fantasy. Occasionally dreaming, poetry and sexual satisfaction are thrown in for good measure.[22] In the normal brain, however, the two hemispheres are united in function as well as in physical fact. Therefore, one must be careful about generalizing too freely from the isolated halves of commissurotomy patients to the integrated brains of normals. Several factors should dampen over-zealous extrapolation to normals.
   First of all, split-brain studies are done with small numbers of individuals, often only one. Thus to generalize a particular finding in one study, one would have to accept that particular individual's left or right hemisphere as representative of everyone's. Clearly this is invalid since each individual is neurologically unique, a point neurologists are careful to make.[23] Split-brain patients are not average individuals and neither of their hemispheres is akin to a normal's. If the epilepsy (which was arrested by the commissurotomy operation) originally arose in the left hemisphere, then there is a good chance that some of the left hemisphere's functions may have

been taken over by the right side. In this case, the right side would be more competent than expected and the left less so. In fact, it is often such reorganization that is of interest, as in the case of P.S.'s communicative right hemisphere. The converse would be true if the original epilepsy was right hemisphere based. Unfortunately, it is impossible to determine the extent of any such transfer.[24] Thus, large numbers of cases are needed for safe generalization, but such large numbers are not available and would present widely varying results anyway.

Another factor increasing the uniqueness of split-brain subjects is the aftermath of the operation itself. Even the surgeon cannot be sure how much of the corpus callosum was cut, how much was spared, or how large the remaining minor commissures are. In addition, some damage is often sustained by one side or the other in the attempt to get at the corpus callosum.

A more serious difficulty with interpreting the results of split brain studies involves the reorganization that occurs *after* the operation. Recall that the right hemisphere dominance for face recognition shown by P.S. only became apparent several months after the operation. If the results of lateralization testing change over time, when should the testing be done?

Pros.   Despite the danger in overgeneralizing from split brain patients, a number of positive arguments can be made. For example, the nontypicality of separated hemispheres can be exploited. With the connections cut, inhibition is also reduced so that even a function for which the hemisphere is nondominant should be expressed to its full extent, i.e. the normally dominant hemisphere will not suppress the activity of the other. In this case, the isolated hemisphere may be giving its best performance. This is not the same as the performance of a normal hemisphere since the interaction between the hemispheres often involves the suppression of one by the other for some activities. Thus, "upper bounds" on performance may be obtained this way.

Split-brain research has been very useful in suggesting avenues for research, because when lateralization differences exist, they are often very dramatic in commissurotomy patients. Having these results to spring from, work with normals, which is invariably less exciting, can be conducted with some sense of certainty. It is fair to say that the dramatic results of hemispheric differences found with split-brain patients in the 1960s provided the enthusiasm for a great deal of the lateralization research conducted since then.

The split-brain model has also proven useful for new approaches to other issues in neuropsychology and psychology. The question of whether or not imaging involves visual processes is one such issue. Similarly, the split-brain model has been applied to the problems of autism and dyslexia.[25] The model may also be used to help conceptualize the difference between verbal and nonverbal thinking, and whether nonverbal intelligence has limits not apparent in our verbal selves. The separation of the mind into verbal and nonverbal halves has already been discussed, and it is clear both sides experience desires, make conclusions, and reflect.

Nonverbal Thinking in Normals. Gazzaniga and LeDoux argue, in introducing their concept of the sociology of mind, that all normals are similar to split-brains in that the two selves within do not communicate completely. This separation would begin in childhood when the corpus callosum is poorly myelinated.[26] During this time, the two selves develop somewhat independently, but in normals one side dominates for certain activities. How is this nonverbal self different from the verbal one? Its strengths are many, perhaps including all the specialties of the right hemisphere. Indeed, on a nonverbal test of intelligence, the right hemispheres of commissurotomy patients did as well or better than the respective left hemispheres.[27] We will discuss this issue of the multiple aspects of personality and possible neurophysiological correlates later in Chapter 14.

NOTES

1. Bogen (1979).
2. Summaries of the split-brain procedure and research can be found in Sperry (1968), Gazzaniga (1970), Gazzaniga & LeDoux (1978) and Bogen (1979).
3. Bogen (1979).
4. Zaidel (1977), Gazzaniga (1970).
5. These results are reviewed by Nebes (1974).
6. Zaidel & Sperry (1973).

7. Ross & Turkewitz (in press).
8. Gazzaniga & LeDoux (1978). As well, when they show that the hemisphere differences disappear with a purely visual task, the scores "ceiling out", that is, they approach or reach 100% for both sides. This may mean that differences between the hemispheres would be detected if the task was made more difficult, because then there would be more room for the scores to vary. The tasks involving copying or tactile identification certainly are difficult enough so that a ceiling effect is not a potential problem.
9. Gazzaniga & Hillyard (1971).
10. These examples are given in Gazzaniga & LeDoux (1978).
11. Gazzaniga & LeDoux (1978, p. 65-66).
12. Gazzaniga (1970). Dennis (1976) argues that the double representation may be due to a lack of callosal inhibition; partial agenesis is more disruptive than complete agenesis in development.
13. Gott & Saul (1978).
14. Risse, LeDoux, Springer, Wilson & Gazzaniga (1978).
15. Gazzaniga & LeDoux (1978, chapter 6).
16. Bogen (1979).
17. Gazzaniga & LeDoux (1978).
18. Bogen (1979, p. 333).
19. Myers (1962).
20. Bogen & Bogen (1969).
21. Ley (1980).
22. See Galin (1976) for a discussion of the metaphors taken too literally.
23. Segalowitz (1980).
24. Whitaker (1978).
25. Zaidel (1979); Kinsbourne (1979). These topics are discussed in more detail in later chapters.
26. The myelin sheath covers the neurons and aids the transmission of the electrical signal. Both physiological evidence (Yakovlev & Lecours, 1967) and behavioral evidence (Galin, Johnstone, Nakell & Herron, 1979) exist for a quite late completion of corpus callosum growth.
27. Zaidel & Sperry (1973) measured nonverbal I.Q. with the Raven's Colored Progressive Matrices Test.

part two

HEMISPHERE ASYMMETRIES IN NORMALS

The great explosion of research in brain lateralization has not only been with clinical populations. The discovery that with some techniques we can detect hemisphere asymmetries in normals has opened the field to many more researchers. The perfecting of these techniques has, in turn, aided the research with patients. In this section, we review these techniques and explore what facets of brain function they reflect. In Chapters 5 and 6, we focus on hemispheric asymmetries for language skills and nonlinguistic functions. The themes raised in these chapters will be repeated throughout the book, as they form the backbone of research in the field.

chapter four

Ways of measuring brain lateralization

Although there is considerable evidence that the two sides of the brain differ in how well they perform certain tasks, all the evidence discussed so far comes from clinical cases. We sometimes refer to these individuals who have suffered brain damage as "natural experiments." By chance, we are provided with examples of brains with various parts missing or damaged. Examination of the abilities of these individuals helps us gain an understanding of how the brain works. Naturally we should not ignore any evidence available to us, but we should be cautious about interpreting it. There are several reasons why we would want to examine normal people who do not have brain damage in order to obtain a more complete idea of the nature of brain lateralization.

First, brain damage is very rarely tidy—bursting blood vessels, bullet wounds, and traffic accidents do not produce clear, localized damage. Even surgery, done for example to relieve epilepsy or to remove a tumor, does not produce clear results because the surgeon removes only as much as is necessary to save the person's life. This amount may overlap two or more structures or may only be part of a structure within the hemisphere. So when we try to make a generalization from left versus right brain-damaged patients, we find each group is far from homogeneous.

A second limitation to cases of brain damage is that we never know how well the person performed before the damage was done, so no comparison can be made. Often this is all right since the deficit is so great that we have no doubt that the person used to be much better at it. For example, the language deficits described in earlier chapters leave no doubt that there has been a loss. However, more subtle distinctions are difficult to make. For these, rather than comparing left and right brain-damaged patients, we would like to compare an individual's intact left hemisphere to his own intact right hemisphere. We might find, for example, that the left hemisphere of most people is better at reading letters than is their right hemisphere, but the reverse is true when matching such shapes as in Figure 4.1. From this we can conclude something fairly firm about the two sides of the brain. Many examples are given in the next chapters about these more subtle differences.

A third reason we should not be satisfied with only evidence from brain damage is that the damage itself may cause changes in the brain functioning that we are interested in. After all, the skill shown by a patient with brain damage is the skill shown by the remaining intact parts of the brain. With a vital component missing, the original balance in the functioning of the brain is lost and a new balance is formed. Although this may be interesting in its own right, generalizations to normals become tricky.

But how can we compare the hemispheres of a normal person without injuring the subject? As discussed in the previous chapter, the input from a number of the senses—especially hearing, vision, and touch—are conveniently lateralized, although not all in the same way. The most popular measures make use of this fact. They are the most popular because the equipment needed for the tests is relatively simple and inexpensive (only by the standards of scientific research!). There are also some other more technically complicated methods of measuring how active each side of the brain is relative to the other, and we will go over these later.

One thing to keep in mind about measuring brain lateralization in intact brains is that since the two halves are well connected, both have access to all information (as is not the case with split-brain

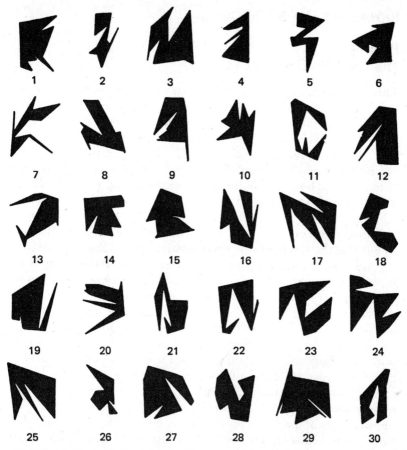

FIGURE 4.1. These random 12-sided figures are the sort that produce a left visual field (right hemisphere) superiority. From Vanderplas & Garvin (1959) "The association value of random shapes." *Journal of Experimental Psychology, 57,* 147–154. Reprinted by permission.

patients). Thus the two sides are going to perform almost identically and any differences will be very small compared to those found with split-brain or brain-damaged patients. With normals, then, we are especially interested in how well each hemisphere performs relative to the other on specific tasks, that is, in the *relative* abilities of each hemisphere.

BEHAVIORAL TECHNIQUES

Hearing:
The Dichotic Listening Task

There is abundant evidence that the two ears are not connected to both hemispheres equally, but that each is more strongly connected to the opposite side. The left ear has *major* connections to the right hemisphere and only *minor* connections to the left hemisphere. For the right ear, the reverse is true. Normally of course, this arrangement has no effect on the person's hearing because both ears receive the same input, so both sides of the brain are amply supplied. Even if you listen with only one ear, as with a telephone for instance, both sides of the brain receive the message because the minor connections are certainly adequate to pass it along. Besides, the corpus callosum connecting the two hemispheres transmits across whatever is heard.

However, interesting things happen when different input is supplied to each ear. First of all, there is some physiological evidence[1] that when both ears receive input, the minor connections that go to the same side of the brain as the ear—called *ipsilateral* pathways—are blocked. So, the message only goes via the major, *contralateral* pathways. If the two ears are hearing the same thing, we experience nothing strange since both sides receive the same message. However, if the messages are different, each side first receives only a single message via the contralateral pathways. The other message must cross by the corpus callosum (see Figure 4.2). This second message is presumed to be weaker because it is coming at a time when the hemisphere is already busy with the other input and also because some information may be lost in the transfer across the corpus callosum. This procedure is called a *dichotic listening* test.

So we have a situation where we can put different information into each hemisphere of a person who is not split-brained. Let us trace what would happen to such input in a person who was left-lateralized for language skills. Say we put the word "one" in the left ear and "two" in the right ear (see Figure 4.3). The "two" would arrive at the language hemisphere first and therefore have a better chance of being understood. We would expect the ear opposite to the language hemisphere to show an advantage over the other ear for recognizing words. People with language represented in the left

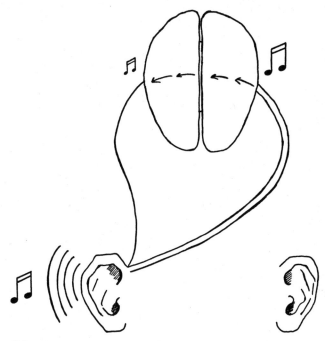

FIGURE 4.2. Each ear is connected to both hemispheres, but the contralateral pathways are larger than the ipsilateral ones. The sound as well gets to the ipsilateral hemisphere by way of the corpus callosum.

hemisphere should show a right ear advantage and those with language in the right hemisphere (a small group, of course) should show a left ear advantage on this task. The difference need not be large, but it should be relatively consistent in a large group of people. This is exactly what Doreen Kimura showed in a classic set of studies in 1961. She showed that patients, who because of Wada testing (see Chapter 2) were known to have left hemisphere language, display a right ear advantage and those with right-hemisphere language display a left ear advantage.

The dichotic listening model is seen clearly in tests with split-brain patients who can easily report what is heard in either ear if presented monaurally. However, there is a dramatic drop in the reports of left ear input with dichotic presentation. With normals,

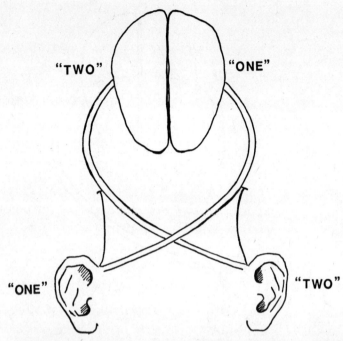

"TWO"   "ONE"

"ONE"   "TWO"

FIGURE 4.3. In the dichotic listening model, the ipsilateral (same-sided) projection is blocked by the contralateral input. Thus, the two inputs cross to the opposite hemispheres, and only then transfer to the other side through the corpus callosum. In the split-brain patient, the left ear input cannot cross, and so goes unreported (by the left hemisphere). In normals the right ear input has an advantage presumably coming from its more direct access to the left hemisphere.

the left ear reports are about 10 percent to 15 percent lower than those of the right ear. In split-brain patients, the left ear reports drop to zero. Presumably in this case, the input goes only to the opposite hemisphere and without the corpus callosum intact, these patients cannot transfer the information from the right hemisphere to the speech areas in the brain.[2]

We don't have to use only digits as stimuli. We can make up dichotic test tapes with pretty well any sounds we like—single sounds, syllables, words of various sorts, environmental sounds such as horns, trains, thunder, music, and so on. The only restriction is that the sounds must be carefully edited to start in each ear simultaneously, end simultaneously, and be of the same loudness.[3] If one hemisphere is superior to the other in processing the stimuli, then we should find an ear advantage on the opposite side. By carefully selecting the sounds used, we can find out what kind of processing each hemisphere is better at. The main selecting feature so far has been the language/nonlanguage distinction that we have already discussed. However, as we will see in the next chapter, many finer distinctions can be made that help us focus on perhaps the primary sources of hemisphere differences.

Vision: The Visual
Half-Field Technique

As we saw in the discussion of research on split-brain patients, the two visual fields (not the two eyes) connect to the opposite hemispheres.[4] The reason was shown in Figure 3.2. We are free to present any visual stimulus we want, but it must be presented very quickly to the visual half-field. This is because the natural reaction is for the subject in the experiment to move his eyes over to focus on the stimulus. If he were allowed to do this, then the stimulus would no longer be in a visual half-field, but now would be in the center, with parts perceived by each hemisphere. The time taken to move one's eyes to focus on something on one side is about one-fifth of a second, so all stimuli must be presented faster than this in order to make sure that they are indeed laterally presented.

The usual procedure is to present a dot centrally as a fixation point so the subject will be looking straight ahead. A stimulus is presented for under 1/5 second (often for less than 1/10 second) to one side or the other, and the subject must respond to it, by naming the object shown or by pushing a button to indicate something about the stimulus, such as whether it was the same or different from another stimulus. If the judgment required takes place primarily in one hemisphere, then the responses to the side opposite to that hemisphere should be more accurate and perhaps also faster. The reasons for this are the same as in the dichotic listening task: the information going to the "wrong" side must either be poorly processed by the inappropriate hemisphere, or the information must be transferred via the corpus callosum to the other side, arriving later and perhaps in damaged condition as well.

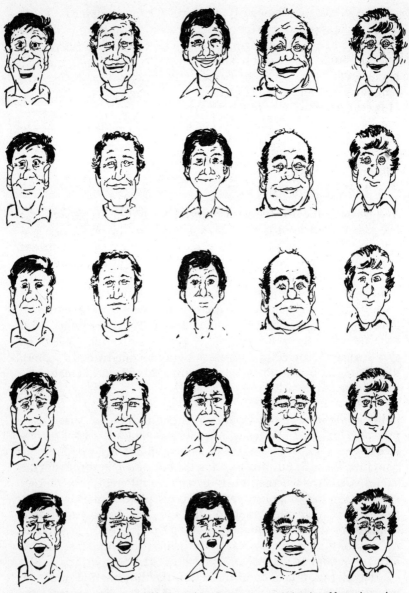

FIGURE 4.4. Identification of the emotional expression and identity of faces is easier in the left visual field than in the right visual field. Ley & Bryden (1979) demonstrated this with the faces reproduced here. Reprinted by permission.

For example, Robert Ley and Phil Bryden[5] presented subjects with cartoon drawings of faces of 5 characters each portraying 5 emotions ranging from very positive to very negative (see Figure 4.4). They first presented one of the 25 drawings laterally to the left or to the right of fixation for 85 milliseconds (thousandths of a second), and then immediately afterwards a second face in the center of the screen. The subject first indicated whether the emotions of the two faces were the same or different, and then whether the character was the same or different. For both judgments, there was a clear superiority when the stimuli were presented in the left visual field. That is, the right hemisphere showed a clear advantage for this task.

Many other types of stimuli have been used with this paradigm, for example, judgments of line orientations, counting of dots, reading of letters and reading of items on clock faces.[6]

Touch: The Dichhaptic Task

One of the earliest known brain asymmetries is the cross-over pattern for motor control and touch perception. Damage to the left side of the brain can cause a right-sided paralysis and loss of sensation. It turns out that not all motor control is lateralized,[7] but as far as we know all touch perception is. In order to exploit this, Sandra Witelson[8] presented a series of approximately 1½ inch square shapes simultaneously to both hands of subjects for identification. If the stimuli were letters of the alphabet, the subject identified the shapes with a verbal response. If they were abstract shapes, the subject responded by picking them out of a collection shown to them (see Figure 4.5). Generally, letters were slightly better identified by the right hand while the shapes were much better recognized when first identified with the left hand. From this, Witelson concluded that this left hand advantage was due to the superiority of the right hemisphere in dealing with spatial tasks, which corroborates what we already know from work with brain damaged and split-brain patients. Conversely, right hand superiority on letter recognition would be due to its more direct link to the language processing hemisphere.

It is not odd that the right hand should be superior in recognizing letters, since the subjects are right handed. The startling aspect of these results is that the left hand should show superior tactual skill at all in *right-handed* people. The direct link to right

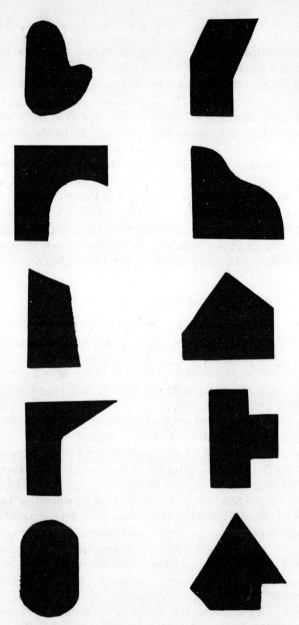

FIGURE 4.5. Witelson (1974) used random shapes such as these in her dichhaptic paradigm and found a left hand superiority for identifying them. Courtesy of S.F. Witelson.

hemisphere skills provides the reason, and also accounts for other startling results similar to these. For example, right-handed people find it easier to read Braille with the left hand[9] and right-handed touch typists make fewer errors with the left hand.[10]

TAPPING BRAIN ACTIVITY

The three sensory modalities discussed provide the main avenues to testing the hemispheres somewhat separately in normal people. Other measures tap more directly into brain functioning by looking at direct correlates of brain activity—electrical patterns as recorded by an electroencephalograph (EEG) and the amount of blood flowing to various regions of the brain.

The EEG record is a pattern of changes in electrical activity in the brain, sometimes called brain waves. A particular pattern is called a *waveform*. An EEG recording is taken by placing electrically sensitive monitors on a person's scalp. The minute electrical signals picked up are on the order of 20 *millionths* of a volt, and are amplified about 20,000 times before they are recorded (see Figure 4.6). The minute signals are the result of the electrical activity of the millions of brain cells below the monitors. The signals from the millions of cells in the region of a particular monitor all contribute to the electrical pattern. The waveform as a result of this is a sum of all the activity within "listening" range of the monitor. There is no way to separate out the effects of nearby brain cells from distant ones, except that nearby ones will have a stronger effect on the EEG because their signals will be picked up better. Some experimental procedures, however, can help us make sense of the signals.

The Average Evoked Response

The EEG signal reflects all the electrical activity of the brain at a particular moment. Naturally the brain is involved in many activities at any one time and it would be naive to think that we could make any firm conclusions by simply looking at one EEG sample from a normal person.

Let us say we want to find a way of reflecting the brain asymmetry for processing words using an EEG record. One favored way is

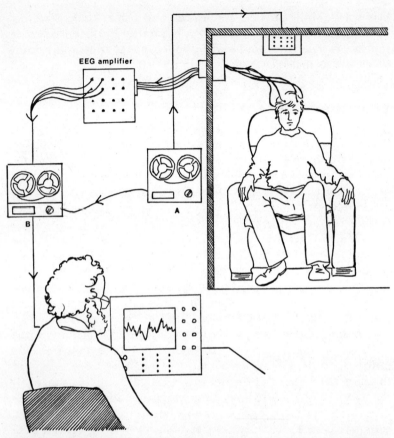

FIGURE 4.6. In an EEG experiment, the subject sits in an electrically shielded cage that blocks other signals, such as 60-cycle electrical interference from the room light, from being recorded. Tape recorder A plays a stimulus to the subject while simultaneously recording it on tape recorder B, which also records the EEG signals. In this way, on tape B the brain wave activity can be linked to specific stimuli such as words or music. The EEG signals must be amplified at least 20,000 times before recording them.

to mark on the recorded EEG exactly each spot when a word is spoken, let us say 50 times. Each of the 50 instances is called an *evoked response* and is a measure of the brain activity during the processing of that word. But the 50 evoked responses all look different! This is because there is a great deal of "noise" in the signal—electrical activity that also reflects the rest of the brain's activity besides the response to hearing the word. Somewhere in each of those evoked responses is the waveform pattern that reflects hearing the word. In order to isolate it, we can average over the 50 evoked responses, producing an *averaged evoked response*, or AER. The AER corresponds to the specific effect of the word because the rest of the signals—the noise—averages out (see Figure 4.7). In one evoked response the electrical signal may be made more positive because of concurrent activity, but the next time it may be more negative. Over a large number of trials, the noise averages out because it is assumed to be random with respect to the onset of the stimulus. All that remains is the consistent pattern produced by the word.

Now, we can examine these consistent patterns from different spots on the scalp, comparing for example AERs from similar areas

FIGURE 4.7. Single auditory evoked responses are an unreliable reflection of the brain response to a sound. An average of 18 responses, however, cancels out much of the noise due to sources other than the auditory event (in this case, a click occurring at the arrow). Averaging over 120 responses produces an even cleaner response.

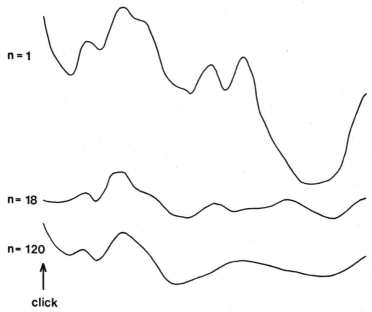

n = 1

n = 18

n = 120

click

on the left side versus right side of the head (see Figure 4.6). There are a number of ways of making these comparisons, including the following three.

Positive and Negative Peaks. One traditional way of comparing two (or more) AERs is to look for specific positive and negative peaks. Remember that the evoked response is an average of electrical responses. It is a waveform of positive and negative movements. The degree of positive and negative changes can be quantified and comparisons made. For example, a positive electrical peak that has brought considerable attention is called P300, because it occurs approximately 300 milliseconds (.3 seconds) after the start of a stimulus. It appears to reflect some measure of attention given to the stimulus. If the P300 is larger on the left side of the head, we would conclude that that side is paying more attention to the stimulus, for whatever reason. For example, the response in the left hemisphere is greater than that in the right when words are seen and vice versa when dot patterns are seen.[11] Interestingly, the stimuli alone do not determine the lateralized response as the asymmetry may shift without changing the items, simply by having the subject treat them differently. For example, when the sound of a speech syllable is identified, a greater left hemisphere response is obtained. When the same syllable is judged for its pitch, no such asymmetry is produced.[12]

Principal Components Analysis. The analysis of positive and negative peaks only looks at a few particular points in the AER waveforms. Clearly, there are many spots that could be examined. The principal components analysis (PCA) is a complicated statistical procedure that makes use of all points on the waveform, keeping track of the relations between the electrical signals at the various points. Thus with this method, rather than finding a relation between two points, the entire shape of the wave pattern is considered. More information in the EEG record is taken into account in this way, allowing for applications beyond tasks that provide an attentional reaction.[13]

Correlations. We may not be interested in the amount of attention paid to stimuli, but rather in how discriminating each side of the brain is. For example, Warren Brown and his colleagues[14] played a tape recording of repetitions of the two sentences "Sit by the fire" and "Ready aim fire" to subjects while making EEG recordings. The actual recording for the word "fire" was identical for both sentences, since they had spliced two copies of the original into the two sentences. In one sentence, the word is a noun, in the other a verb.

Instead of looking for positive and negative peaks, they wanted to see whether the AERs from each side of the head for the noun and verb form were similar or different. The statistical measure is called a *correlation coefficient*. The higher this number is, with a maximum of 1.0, the more similar these two AERs are. A correlation of zero means there is no relationship. What Brown, Marsh & Smith found was that the left side produced low correlations between the noun and verb forms (averages were .07 for the front and .19 for the back of the head) while they were high on the right side (averages were .79 for the front and .84 for the back). Thus the left side seems to make more of a distinction between the noun and verb forms while the right side doesn't. Perhaps the right side only processed the word "fire" as a sound, not as a word with grammatical and contextual meaning.

EEG Alpha Asymmetry

A limitation of AER analysis is that only short segments, about one second long at most, can be analyzed and the stimulus must be presented many times for averaging. Clearly there are mental activities that we may want to investigate that take longer than one second and cannot be repeated. For example, finding a solution to a jigsaw puzzle takes more than one second and once the solution is discovered, the puzzle cannot be used again. An alternative way to analyze the EEG record is to look for organized, somewhat slow patterns. Of special interest is a pattern called *alpha waves* (see Figure 4.8). When this type of signal is generated, the brain is resting. Concentrated thinking, figuring, and problem solving generate what looks like very "fast wave" activity, called beta waves. This is because the brain cells are busy in many mental operations. Such active thinking generally reduces alpha waves.

We can use this phenomenon to test for differences in how active each hemisphere is during a particular task, by seeing which shows less alpha. For example, Robert Ornstein and David Galin[15]

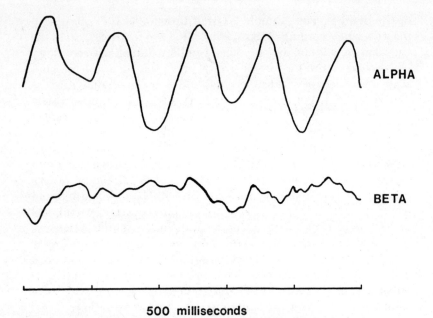

500 milliseconds

FIGURE 4.8. Alpha waves (8 to 13 cycles per second) are used as an indication of a relative lack of active thinking (and often appear when the subject is bored and drowsy, as in the excerpt above). Beta activity, on the other hand, indicates active processing, as in the above example where the same subject attended to the task once more.

found greater alpha in the left hemisphere while subjects did two spatial tasks and greater alpha in the right hemisphere while verbal tasks were done. Keeping in mind that alpha is an indication of *less* organized thinking, their results conform to our expectations.

The benefit of using relative alpha as an indicator of brain lateralization is that subjects can perform tasks as they normally would. The measure is not restricted to short, time-linked activities as in the AER.

Regional Cerebral Blood Flow (CBF)

When brain cells fire impulses, electrical fields are established, which are reflected in the EEG record. With each cell firing, some specific chemicals are used up. The electrical impulse is not a flow of electrons as in an electric wire, but rather a chemical chain reaction. In order to fire again, these chemicals must be replaced. The source for these chemical nutrients is the blood supply, which can be amazingly specific in its delivery system. By measuring the amount of blood supplying various parts of the brain during special activities, we can see which part of the brain is most active during those activities.

The primary way[16] of measuring blood flow in the brain is by having the subject inhale an inert gas with a very low-level radioactive tracer. This tracer can then be followed and the path charted on a diagram of the brain. For example, during a resting state, there appears to be a high level of activity in the frontal lobes, but when speaking occurs, the left hemisphere language areas become active (see Figure 4.9). This is clearly a useful tool for examing a patient's cerebral blood flow, for example to check for blood clots or burst vessels. Also, however, this system can help us determine which brain areas are most active during specific types of thinking.

Another approach, which is also built on the idea that blood flow reflects brain activity, involves just a left versus right hemi-

FIGURE 4.9. Measurements of cerebral blood flow reflect the activation of brain tissue in different parts of the cortex. Here we see that during talking, compared to a resting state, there is an increase in temporal lobe activity. From Ingvar (1976). Reprinted by permission.

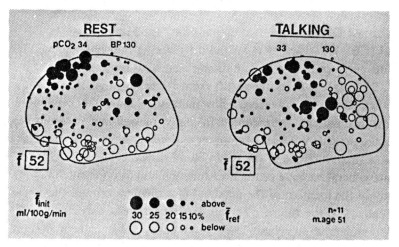

sphere comparison. James Dabbs[17] has measured very minute differences in the temperature of each side, presumably reflective of the blood flow. The differences, measured in 100ths of a degree, were recorded during a resting state. Right-handed subjects with high verbal and low spatial abilities had a greater flow on the left; high spatial-low verbal subjects had more flow on the right.

Electrodermal Asymmetry

The electrical and blood flow changes in the brain are reflections of changes in brain activity. The electrical resistance of the skin is also an indirect reflection of brain activity, with a rise in conductance during higher arousal and emotional reactions. The lie detector is based on this principle. In addition, however, the skin conductance can be measured separately for each hand while the subject is performing various tasks, such as verbal versus visual-spatial activities. In such an experiment, right-handed subjects have significantly greater right hand skin conductance on a verbal task compared with either a simple tone or light presentation (these control situations produced no asymmetry), while a greater left hand skin conductance is produced during a visual imagery task.[18]

MOMENTUM AND INERTIA

All the measures of lateralization discussed so far have made use of either input and output asymmetries or direct physiological correlates of brain activity. There is another that makes use of the notion that brain activity builds up momentum and inertia just like any other activity. There are two ways of taking advantage of such activity, the first by using the momentum, the other by using the inertia.

Lateral Eye Movements (LEMs)

If one area of the brain is especially more active than the other at a particular time, then it is possible that the activity "spills over" to other brain areas near the active sites. This is called a "general activation" model. In other words, the electrical activity of one area can induce activity nearby. One activity that might be affected by such overflow is the movement of the eyes. There is not much reason to move the eyes one way or the other while thinking if you are looking at a perfectly symmetrical (or blank) wall. Thus, if there is any overflow at all, it might be detected in lateral eye movements.[19] LEMs are driven by impulses from the contralateral hemisphere—left movements are due to innervation arising in the right hemisphere, right movements from the left hemisphere. Thus, while thinking of something that requires primarily left hemisphere activity, for example thinking of a word with four *i*'s in it, the eye gaze should move toward the right. However, there must be no other motivation to look left or right, nothing to look at, no noises, no asymmetric lighting.[20] Such conditions are sometimes difficult to produce, and the LEM test is often far from reliable as a measure of hemisphere activation.[21] However, the advantage of LEMs as a lateralization test is obvious: Any task can be performed while eye movements are charted.

Concurrent Manual Tasks

Continuing with the analogy of movement, the tendency for the brain to continue along a particular path of activity and to find competing responses to be distracting can be likened to inertia. If we accept the general activation model outlined in the previous section, then it follows that uncoordinated activations in two nearby areas can interfere with each other. For example, if one recites a poem and simultaneously tries to tap a finger not in rhythm with the speaking, there should be interference. The interference should be reduced by tapping a finger not controlled by the hemisphere that is busy with the speaking. The converse, of course, should also be found and it is—reciting a nursery rhyme disrupts finger tapping with the right hand more than with the left hand.[22] Similar results are found with more complicated manual tasks, such as sequentially tapping four telegraph keys with different fingers[23] or balancing a dowel on the end of a finger.[24]

Do the Tests
Measure the Same Thing?

With all these ways of detecting brain asymmetries, we can legitimately ask whether they reflect the same thing. After all, they make use of different sense modalities and different kinds of responses. We will leave until Chapter 15 a more detailed discussion of some of the difficulties involved in using and interpreting the measures. However, different researchers do not always agree on what is lateralized in the human brain and some of this disagreement may be attributable to the differences in the tasks. For example, the dichotic listening task requires listening skills and good auditory memory. The visual half-field technique, on the other hand, requires visual attention and often visual recognition with a minimum of memory. If we are interested in lateralization for language processing, which test should we use? It would probably be best to use both, but the results from both do not always agree with each other [25] and it is time consuming to do both tasks. The safest approach is to try to find studies that use various tests but are aiming at the same research question. For example, which hemisphere is superior in understanding abstract words? This can be tested with almost all the techniques described. If the various tests produce the same result, we can be fairly sure it is correct and not due to some artifact of a particular test. This approach is called *triangulation* and is common in experimental psychology when researchers examine unseen, abstract processes.

The Meaning of "Lateralization"

So far we have been discussing brain lateralization as if it referred to only one thing. But it should be clear by now that the various pieces of evidence from brain-damaged patients, from split-brain patients, and from the many tasks with normals probably reflect different aspects of brain functioning. Comparing various studies, it is clear the term "lateralization" is interpreted a number of ways.[26] Keeping these distinctions in mind may help sort out some of the complexities. Consider the following three.

Hemispheric Competence.   How good is each hemisphere at a particular task? This is usually what we mean by "lateralization," but in order to test each hemisphere independently they must be separated. This is only possible in split-brain patients. Tests with normals are often interpreted as if they were tests of competence, but they really are not.

Hemispheric Dominance. Which hemisphere controls the input and output? Which hemisphere is the "executive?" We would normally expect the most competent hemisphere to be dominant for the function. Certainly this would be most efficient, but is not always the case, as we saw in Chapter 3 in the evidence from split-brain cases. In studies with normals, a superior performance by one side may reflect either superior competence or a dominance by one hemisphere.

Hemispheric Participation. Does a particular brain region contribute to the work being done? This is a measure of activity, not competence nor dominance. The EEG and the cerebral blood flow (CBF) techniques reflect degrees of activity. However, a brain region or hemisphere can participate—for example, show reduced alpha waves or increased blood flow—without being dominant or even highly competent for the task.

With these various meanings in mind, we can rephrase many of the fascinating questions to be more precise. For example, "Does lateralization relate to ability?" becomes, "Is overall ability in a task related to degree of asymmetric competence, degree of dominance by one side, or degree of asymmetric participation?" "Do different personality types have different lateralization?" becomes, "Are different personality types associated with differences in asymmetry of competence, degree of dominance by one side, or degree of asymmetric participation?" It is usually the middle interpretation (dominance) that is intended (see Chapter 11).

Although these distinctions are correct and useful conceptually, they are not so clear in practice. An asymmetry on a visual half field task, for instance, may be due to any or all of the three. Although I will try to be as specific as possible in the following chapters concerning the meaning of "lateralization," the state of the art is such that a certain vagueness is unavoidable.

NOTES

1. Rosenzweig (1951), Hall & Goldstein (1968), Aitken & Webster (1972).
2. Kimura (1961a,b); Sparks & Geschwind (1968).

3. See Berlin & Cullen (1977) and Berlin & McNeil (1976) for a detailed discussion of the variables involved in making up a dichotic listening tape. See also Gruber & Segalowitz (1977) for a discussion of some complications in interpreting results.
4. Blakemore (1970), Mitchell & Blakemore (1969), Gazzaniga (1970, pp. 90–94).
5. Ley & Bryden (1979).
6. Kimura (1969), Levy & Reid (1976), and Davidoff (1977), but see Bryden (1976); Cohen (1972), Segalowitz & Stewart (1979); Berlucchi, Brizzolara, Marzi, Rizzolatti & Umilta (1979).
7. Fine movements are controlled only contralaterally; for gross movements there is some bilateral control (Brinkman & Kuypers, 1972).
8. Witelson (1974). See Gazzaniga & LeDoux (1978, pp. 29–39) for a discussion of lateralized representation of active versus passive touch.
9. Hermalin & O'Connor (1971); Rudel, Denckla & Spalten (1974).
10. Provins & Glencross (1968).
11. Buchsbaum & Fedio (1969).
12. Wood, Goff & Day (1971).
13. For examples of applications see Chapman, Bragdon, Chapman & McCrary (1977), Molfese (1979).
14. Brown, Marsh & Smith (1973, 1976).
15. Ornstein & Galin (1976), Galin & Ornstein (1972), Galin (1978), Moore & Haynes (1980).
16. Lassen, Ingvar & Skinhoj (1978); Wood (1980); Ingvar (1976); Risberg & Ingvar (1973).
17. Dabbs (1980); Dabbs & Choo (1980).
18. Myslobodsky & Rattok (1977).
19. Kinsbourne (1972); Kinsbourne & Hicks (1978).
20. Kinsbourne (1974).
21. Ehrlichman & Weinberger (1978).
22. Hiscock & Kinsbourne (1978); Kinsbourne & Cook (1971); Rizzolatti, Bertoloni & Buchtel (1979).
23. Lomas & Kimura (1976).
24. Kinsbourne & Cook (1971).
25. Bryden (1965); Fennell, Bowers & Satz (1977).
26. Galin (1979).

chapter five

Lateralization for language functions

As mentioned earlier, in Chapter 1, the predominance of the left hemisphere for language skills earned for that side the attribution of "dominant hemisphere." Despite John Hughlings Jackson's early prediction that the right side would eventually be found to be superior in certain perceptual skills, the prestige of the left hemisphere continued to rise.[1] By the early part of this century, the notion of the left side being dominant for language had spread to include virtually all intellectual skills, so that some even claimed that no particular symptoms follow from right hemisphere damage, and that the right hemisphere's function is to wait and serve the other side if and when needed.

This is now clearly inadequate as a description of the right hemisphere's role. However, the degree of functional advantage for the left side is greatest for language related behaviors. In this chapter, we will discuss the linguistic skills that lend so much status to the left hemisphere, and explore what it may be that underlies the representation of verbal processing in the left cerebral hemisphere.

From the study of aphasia, it is obvious that in most people, the left hemisphere is crucial for language use. Yet it is not obvious why this is so, what it is about the left side that makes it dominant for language skills. Later, we will explore some of the possibilities. First, we should note that for normals, there is also overwhelming evidence that ordinary language use emphasizes left-side participation. In other words, not only is the left hemisphere crucial for some aspect of language, it is also more active overall in the process. This has been demonstrated with three paradigms suitable for examining hemisphere activity during an ongoing task.

David Galin and Robert Ornstein measured the relative amount of alpha wave output from each side while subjects were composing a letter and when they were manipulating shapes. Each task type was done twice, once mentally and once physically. For example, subjects mentally composed a letter and then actually wrote it. In each case, the letter writing task produced greater alpha over the right hemisphere than over the left (remember that alpha reflects the degree of *non*participation in the task) compared to manipulating the shapes.[2]

Similarly, a number of researchers have found that a manual task requiring fine motor control is more disrupted on the right by speaking than on the left.[3] Eye movements to the right also seem to be more likely than movements to the left when the subject is solving a verbal problem as opposed to a visual-spatial problem.[4]

As compelling as all these studies are, we are still left with the question of why a language task involves primarily left hemisphere processes. Language is a multifaceted skill. Let us examine what contribution each facet makes to the overall lateralization of language.

Components of Language

Since we use language rather automatically every day, we are not aware of the many processes needed for construction of the simplest sentence. For a scientific study, we should examine more carefully what it is that makes up linguistic skill. The divisions that are now generally accepted include these four:

1. The processing of speech sounds (phonology): dealing with and producing the sounds of the language. A *phoneme* is an abstrac-

tion of a sound unit in a language. Despite variations in the final product, we have some ideal version of speech sounds in mind when we listen or talk. Phonemes differ from one language to another and even from one region to another, producing local accents. Even within one individual, a particular phoneme may have variants—such as the vowel sound in "half" and "have" where the length is considerably longer in the second word, or the *p*-sound in "spit" versus "pit," where the amount of breath (aspiration) varies considerably.

2. The processing of the rules of grammar (syntax): the rules of word order and word form, generally referred to as "grammar" in public school.

3. The processing of meaning (semantics): the meanings of words in isolation and in combination. The division between semantics and syntax is sometimes rather fine, since the grammatical structure of a sentence is often dependent on the meanings of the words in it.

4. Pragmatics: This category is a grab bag of facets of language not included in the other categories, such as intonation and speech acts (see Chapter 2).

It should be clear that these four aspects of language use are interdependent (e.g. by changing the intonation pattern, one can turn a statement into a question), and some linguists and psychologists may prefer other divisions or groupings. For example, it is very difficult at times to judge whether a certain linguistic distinction is due to syntactic or semantic aspects. Yet for our purposes, this four-way division will be useful in examining brain lateralization effects in language processing.

Phonology: the Processing of Speech Sounds. In the dichotic listening test, which is probably the best known and most accepted task reflecting brain lateralization, Doreen Kimura originally employed pairs of digits or words for identification, one for each ear. Generally, digits or words played to the right ear are better identified than those played to the left ear. However, the digits used—the numbers *1* to *9* excluding *7* (the only one with two syllables)—are relatively recognizable and discriminable. How much of the relative scores for each side is due to recognition of sounds *per se*, compared with the hemispheres' knowledge of the meaning of each word or ability to reconstruct what the word must be from only a fragment that is heard? In order to get at "pure" word recognition, where all the subject can do is make sense of the sounds, Donald Shankweiler and Michael Studdert-Kennedy presented nonsense syllables consisting of a consonant-vowel-consonant (CVC) combination or simply a consonant-vowel (CV) combination. They used the consonants *b*, *d*, *g*, *p*, *t*, *k*, and 6 vowels *ee*, *e*, *a*, *ah*, *o*, and *oo*. For the CVC stimuli, the consonant *p* provided the end consonant for one experiment and provided the initial sound for a second study.

In these experiments, although the listeners might know that only twelve sounds are used, they could not predict which combinations will appear. Shankweiler and Studdert-Kennedy found that initial consonants produced the greatest right ear advantage (indicating the most left hemisphere bias) the final consonants less of a bias, and the vowels no bias at all.[5] Thus all speech sounds do not produce an identical left hemisphere bias. One way of explaining these differences is by examining the sounds used. It turns out that the consonants used in their studies provide a complex pattern of sounds, especially when they are in the initial position. These sounds involve a rapid change in the structure of the sound (called *transitions*), while the vowels do not (hence they are called *steady state vowels*). The changes are of very short duration, on the order of thousandths of a second, but are absolutely necessary for identifying the consonants. The sounds with transitions are referred to as *encoded* speech sounds, while the others are not.[6] Thus it is suggested that the left hemisphere is required for understanding encoded speech.

Is this enough to account for language dominance in the brain? No, because steady state vowels can be made to produce a right ear advantage when the task is made more difficult.[7] As well, there are other cues associated with greater left-hemisphere involvement, including whether or not the sounds are *thought* of as speech. When subjects think of vowel segments as humming, the right ear advantage disappears. When Thai speakers are given a dichotic listening task where they must identify tone inflections in their language, a right ear advantage is found, while subjects who don't know Thai produce no advantage.[8] Thus, there are probably many other factors besides speech encoding that favor the left hemisphere. It is true, though, that a healthy left hemisphere is necessary for identifying speech sounds. Patients with left-sided damage have difficulty identifying speech sounds.[9]

All this evidence that the left hemisphere is prepotent for speech sound discrimination does not mean that the right hemisphere is passive during the task. On the contrary, EEG records show almost identical processing in the two hemispheres, with some of the speech cues discriminated better in the left hemisphere (such as transitions), while others are dealt with possibly even more in the right hemisphere, such as *voice onset time*, which distinguishes *b,d,* and *g* from *p,t,* and *k* respectively.[10] Note here the distinction raised in the last chapter between *dominance* and *participation.* The EEG data concern only how involved the hemisphere is in the activity and in making certain discriminations. On the other hand, dichotic listening tasks tap dominance, the degree of control over input and output. Thus, the right ear advantage traditionally found for discriminating CV syllables (especially the commonly used *ba, pa, da, ta, ga,* and *ka* comparisons) reflects an aspect of lateralization different from the EEG data on voice onset time. Left-hemisphere dominance does not preclude right hemisphere participation in the task.

Thus, the left hemisphere is dominant for the reception and production of speech (as discussed in Chapter 2). Left brain-damaged patients have difficulty with phonological discriminations, to be sure, yet the right side may be crucial for some nonlinguistic acoustic processing, that is, some sound discriminations not limited to language use. Such possibilities will be explored further in the next chapter.

Syntax: The Processing of Grammar.   Clearly, the proper use of grammar is disrupted in aphasia. Yet, the improper use of syntax in aphasia may be due to disruption of other components of the language system. For example, if some words are mistaken for others that sound similar or mean something else, then no doubt the patient will seem to have lost the use of grammatical rules as well. Recall the excerpts of aphasic speech given in Chapter 2. Despite this confounding of language aspects in aphasia, there is really no question about which hemisphere is dominant for grammatical disruption, despite some other related losses. In the aphasia literature, a more critical issue is whether or not there is a loss of grammatical knowledge in Broca's aphasia, caused by frontal lobe damage.[11] For a more precise demonstration of the link between specific grammatical processing and the left hemisphere, we must turn to experiments with normals.

In normals, the dichotic listening and evoked response paradigms have been applied to the question of lateralization of grammatical functions. For example, when sentences made up of nonsense words (e.g. "The wak jud shendily") are presented dichotically, a right ear advantage ensues. When the aspects that make it sound like a sentence are removed—for example, by reading the words in a "laundry list" fashion and with the word endings rearranged to disrupt the implication of subject-predicate ordering—the right ear advantage is lost.[12] On a finer scale, recall the study in the previous chapter, in which evoked response recordings from the left and right hemispheres reflect more participation by the left side in the distinction between the two grammatical uses of a word ("Sit by the *fire*" versus "Ready, aim, *fire*"). In this study, the identical strip of recording tape was used for each meaning, indicating that the differentiation was due to grammatical use of the word rather than any change in sound. As described in the last chapter, what the researchers found was that the average evoked EEG response over the right hemisphere was substantially the same for each use of the word, while the left side differentiated between them.[13]

Semantics: The Understanding of Word Meanings. The proper use of word meanings is grossly disrupted in the posterior aphasias, such as Wernicke's. No known syndrome involving only the right hemisphere produces similar effects on the use of appropriate word meaning. Yet it could be that in specific cases, the degree of left hemisphere dominance for the understanding of words is lessened. This may be because the right hemisphere is not totally ignorant of some words as sounds or as visual symbols. For example, some words are more abstract, others more concrete. The more concrete ones are more imageable, such as *chair* or *cloud*, compared to abstract nouns as *truth* or *hate*. Are the more imageable ones more readily understood and coded in the right hemisphere? The answer is yes. For example, when abstract and concrete words were presented in a dichotic listening paradigm, the right ear (left hemisphere) was more accurate in identifying the abstract items. The left ear (right hemisphere) was better on the concrete words.[14] Similarly, in a visual half-field paradigm, the left hemisphere bias in reading abstract words is greater than that for concrete words.[15]

A similar hemisphere difference is suggested for emotional versus nonemotional words. It has long been known that aphasics who seem to have lost all speech can occasionally produce impressive outbursts of oaths if highly aroused.[16] Recall Ley's study described in Chapter 3. Following up on this observation, he found that in normals trying to remember emotion-laden words, either positive (as *hero* or *love*) or negative (as *cancer* or *corpse*), tend to activate the right hemisphere compared to remembering neutral words. In his study, left ear accuracy increased when emotional words were being remembered.[17] Presumably it is the meanings of these words that produce the asymmetries, and so it would seem that emotional words encourage an increase in right hemisphere control.

Note that the conclusion of right hemisphere involvement in the coding of certain types of words is a speculative leap from the data. In the dichotic listening study and in Robert Ley's work just mentioned, it is the *memory* of certain words that alters the usual hemisphere asymmetry. Therefore, it may be the meaning itself rather than the symbol (i.e. the word) that involves right hemisphere processes. Also, the notion of the right side being worse for abstract notions than for concrete words runs counter to the general finding that right hemisphere-damaged patients tend to be overly concrete. They are less able, with a malfunctioning right hemisphere, to deal with abstractions such as metaphors (see Chapter 2).

A major problem with testing the right hemisphere for word meaning is that while meanings may be accessible by that part of the brain,[18] the task of decoding the symbol for it may require left hemisphere processes. This is dramatically seen in some cases of Japanese aphasics (with left-sided brain damage). There are two writing systems in Japanese, one derived from the Chinese system in which a complex symbol represents the sound of a syllable without any meaning. One system (called *Kanji*) is meaning-based while the other (called *Kana*) is sound-based. Many Japanese aphasics retain some ability to read Kanji words while not being able to read Kana words, producing a situation where the patient selectively reads the Kanji words in a newspaper story.[19] In normals, it has been shown that reading Kana, as with English words, produces a right visual field (left hemisphere) superiority while the Kanji forms show a left visual field (right hemisphere) bias.[20] As far as we know, Kanji words are not more concrete and Kana more abstract. If this were so, the hemispheric difference could be attributed to that dimension.[21] The nature of the writing system, then, can influence the apparent localization of words, the sound-based words being tied to left-hemisphere processes to a greater extent. What this shows is that word meanings may be fairly well dealt with by the right hemisphere, but with its traditional disadvantage in decoding words, whatever skill it has is masked.

Even with English speakers, though, there is considerable room for variation. Not everyone uses exactly the same strategy for reading. Our schools, in fact, fluctuate between two teaching methods, phonics and whole-word. Although most people use a phonics approach to reading at least to some extent, it is conceivable that some people can make do with just recognizing the shape of the words. For example, Ken Heilman reports a case of a right-handed man who suffered a left hemisphere stroke. He became globally aphasic, yet could read quite well (considering his condition). Heilman writes:

> After his discharge, his wife noted that when he wished to communicate what he wanted for dinner he would open a cookbook, read through the references, and indicate what he wanted to eat by pointing to the appropriate place in the text. His wife stated that, in addition to the cookbook, the patient kept other printed material next to his favorite chair and would communicate with her by using this strategy . . . [This patient] was able to learn more than 100 American Indian signs. American Indian signs are a pantomime-based system of gestural communication in which hand postures and motions represent iconic images of major lexical items. With [a subsequent] right hemisphere lesion, the patient lost not only the ability to read but also the ability to comprehend and express these ideographic signs.[22]

Usually, global aphasics are unable to read, but this may be because most (English speaking) readers use a code that is primarily phonics based.

Pragmatics and Other Less Obvious Language Skills. Pronunciation, syntax, and semantics may account for the basic mechanics of language use, but there is much more to communication than this. Even if we could program a computer to deal successfully with the grammar and pronunciation of English, we would find much lacking in its robot-like discourse. Required as well are intonation patterns that subtly reflect the attitude and intent of the speaker. Basic knowledge of the world would be lacking. For example, it would not know that watering the garden and watering the horses are quite different activities. To what extent do these other factors involve lateralized processes?

The ability to use and discriminate intonation patterns and the emotional tone of a sentence clearly involves right hemisphere activity. As was discussed in Chapter 2, aphasics can still discriminate the purpose of an utterance, be it a statement, question, or command. Rather, it is nonaphasic right-hemisphere patients who exhibit a flat intonation and seem to find difficult the determination of the emotional intent of the speaker. Analogous results have been found with normals. When sentences made up of nonsense words are given an intonation contour, there is a left ear (right hemisphere) advantage for identification of that contour, such as telling whether they are declarative, imperative, conditional or interrogative patterns.[23]

Without repeating the discussion of right-hemisphere involvement in language given in Chapter 2, we should remember that many linguistic activities require a healthy right hemisphere. Another example involves the learning of new word meanings. Murray Grossman and Susan Carey tried teaching patients with various types of brain damage a new word, "bice," which refers to the color blue-green. By using it in a series of instructions, such as "Give me the bice pen, not the brown pen," they found that right damaged patients did not seem to appreciate the information implied in such statements—that bice is not brown and that it is a color.[24] This suggests that the right side as well as the left is involved in appreciating the meaning of words in some situations. With normals, an equivalence of the two sides of the brain has been demonstrated for the understanding of relationships. Heeschen and Jurgens gave subjects three-word strings in a dichotic listening paradigm, each string consisting of two nouns and a verb. Proper syntactic structure would be noun-verb-noun, and half the stimulus strings were so ordered (called structured strings). The other half had word orders that were grammatically incorrect, with a verb-noun-noun order (unstructured strings). Right ear (left hemisphere) responses improved when the strings were well structured. Left ear (right hemisphere) responses did not. Thus, the left hemisphere distinguishes and makes use of grammatical structuring. Heeschen and Jurgens also varied the "pragmatic-semantic" value of the pseudo-sentences: In a structured value, the first noun is more likely to be the agent of the verb action, while the second noun is more likely to be the object of the action. For example, a string structured both syntactically and pragmatically would be "Doctor Examine Patient." A syntactically correct but pragmatically unstructured string would have no bias in the relationship, such as in "Gardner Blackmail Youth." Both the left ear and right ear scores improved with pragmatic-semantic structuring, both to the same degree.[25] Thus both hemispheres seemed to take advantage of the structuring of meaning. In some way, then, the right hemisphere makes use of meaning and knowledge, although it is severely handicapped when the information is verbal.

Language and the Left Hemisphere

From what we have covered, it is clear that there are phonological, syntactic, and some semantic factors all favoring left hemisphere representation of language. It is as if there were a conspiracy linking the left side to many of the components necessary for language use. This may be a reflection of a biologically efficient process—making use of skills represented in the same hemisphere to construct a communication system—or an evolutionary process—the converging of just those skills used in language behavior into the left hemisphere.

NOTES

1. Benton (1977), Clarke & Dewhurst (1972).
2. Galin & Ornstein (1972).
3. See Lomas & Kimura (1976), McFarland & Ashton (1978), Hiscock & Kinsbourne (1980), Johnson & Kozma (1977) for a variety of tasks including sequential finger tapping, alternat-

ing index finger movements, tapping with a single finger, and balancing a dowel on one finger, respectively.

4. Kinsbourne (1974); see Erlichman & Weinberger (1978) for a critical review.

5. Shankweiler & Studdert-Kennedy (1967), Studdert-Kennedy & Shankweiler (1970).

6. See Liberman, Cooper, Shankweiler & Studdert-Kennedy (1967) for a summary of the arguments.

7. Such as being uncertain of vocal tract size (Darwin, 1971, 1974) and when a more confusable stimulus set or noise is added to impede perception (Godfrey, 1974).

8. Spellacy & Blumstein (1970); Van Lancker & Fromkin (1973).

9. Zurif & Ramier (1972).

10. See Molfese (1978a) for lateralization for transitions, and Molfese (1978b) for voice onset time processing. A similar argument is given in Ades (1974). We return to these issues in Chapter 12.

11. Zurif & Caramazza (1976); Samuels & Benson (1979).

12. Zurif & Sait (1970), Zurif & Mendelsohn (1972).

13. Brown, Marsh & Smith (1973).

14. In this extension of the traditional dichotic listening paradigm, McFarland, McFarland, Bain & Ashton (1978) had subjects remember a long list of words each presented to one ear or the other. In this case, identifying a word meant correctly indicating whether or not it had been presented before in the list.

15. Hines (1977). See Bradshaw (1980) for a detailed discussion of this work.

16. Van Lancker (1972) reports equal ear advantage for "automatic" speech: stereotyped expressions, brief commands, taboo and swear words.

17. Ley (1980a).

18. There is some evidence that "grammatical meaning," such as differentiating the subject of an action from the object of the action, is treated similarly in the two hemispheres (Segalowitz & Hansson, 1979).

19. Sasasuma (1975), Yamadori (1975).

20. Sasasuma, Itoh, Mori & Kobayashi (1977). See also Hatta (1977). See Segalowitz, Bebout & Lederman (1979) for further discussion on reading symbols and lateralization.

21. At least this is what Park & Arbuckle (1977) found for Korean, which has a similar dual-writing system.
22. Heilman, Rothi, Campanella & Wolfson (1979).
23. Blumstein & Cooper (1974).
24. Grossman & Carey (1978).
25. Heeschen & Jurgens (1977). See also Segalowitz & Hansson (1979) for a similar finding in the visual modality.

chapter six

Nonlinguistic functions

It may seem unjust to devote a whole chapter to linguistic functions and only one of about the same size to nonlinguistic activities. After all, the span of activities in this group is negatively defined, and therefore is theoretically infinite. But in the field of brain lateralization, research on language activities has been overwhelmingly predominant. It is only in the last decade or so that nonlanguage activities have been seriously studied. This imbalance has, of course, contributed to the view that the left hemisphere is more important in all intellectual functions. However, championing the cause of the underdog, a number of neuropsychologists in the last ten years, with all the enthusiasm of explorers charting newly discovered territory, have decried this depreciation of the right side. Many of the nonlanguage activities discussed in this chapter are favored by the right side. For convenience, they will be reviewed under the headings of *auditory effects, emotional factors,* and *visual effects.*

Auditory Effects

Shortly after the dichotic listening test became established as a correlate of dominance for speech, a number of researchers wondered whether the opposite results would appear with nonverbal sounds. It was suggested that environmental noises such as the sounds produced by a racing car, a train, a dripping tap, and so on would produce a left ear (right hemisphere) advantage, and indeed this was the case.[1] Similarly, some nonverbal vocal sounds such as crying, shrieking and laughing are better recognized in the left ear, implying a right hemisphere bias.[2] Is it simply the case that the left hemisphere is better for speech related sounds—even for speech played backward, which many subjects thought sounded vaguely like a Slavic language[3]—and the right side is a grab bag for everything else? Even if we say yes to this rather simple dichotomy, we still must try to find out what it is about speech and nonspeech that cues the hemispheres to the distinction. We will discuss the possibilities after outlining a few more lateralized auditory effects.

Music. Music is often contrasted with language as a highly structured, meaning-endowed yet nonverbal system. As discussed in Chapter 2, some musical functions remain after speech is disrupted in aphasia. More generally, there seems to be a right hemisphere bias for processing music, in terms of hemisphere participation, dominance, and competence as defined in Chapter 4. For example, there is greater relative increase in blood flow in the right hemisphere when patients listen to music (in this case, classical guitar), compared with when they listen to speech.[4] Similarly, the amount of EEG alpha recorded over the right side compared to the left decreases—indicating greater activation—when subjects sing or whistle compared to just speaking the words to a song.[5,6] In this last study, the hemisphere difference was found for nonmusicians only, implying that trained musicians do not engage in the same processes during musical tasks. This is presumably due to the more structured approach to musical tasks that training provides, a difference between musicians and nonmusicians often employed to account for apparent differences in hemispheric bias.

The issue of hemispheric *competence* for music was dealt with in Chapter 2 in the discussion of the dramatic loss of singing skill when the right hemisphere is removed or is temporarily anaesthetized during the Wada test. This contrasts with left-sided damage or incapacitation, which does not seem to affect the ability to carry a tune. Similarly, the ability to use appropriate intonation in ordinary speech also seems to vary with right hemisphere integrity. These cases indicate that it is the right hemisphere alone that is competent for musical patterns. Yet, it is curious that split-brain patients do not show a lack of intonation contour in their speech nor a marked loss of singing skill. Although this has not been studied systematically, it seems reasonable to expect such a loss when the speaking left hemisphere is cut off from the right hemisphere.[7] The lack of such evidence, even anecdotally, suggests that either the left side does in fact harbor some competence or that the corpus callosum is not required for the transfer of the needed information (i.e., the anterior commissure may be adequate). This seeming contradiction between the hemispherectomy and Wada test patients on the one hand and the split-brain patients on the other has yet to be explained.

Hemispheric *dominance* for music and related phenomena such as intonation contour has been demonstrated repetitively by use of the dichotic listening task. Doreen Kimura found that whereas speech sounds (digits) produce a right ear (left hemisphere) advantage, the identification of melodies favors the left ear (right hemisphere).[8] In the same way, so does identification of intonation contour, even when it is in a verbal context.[9] However, music perception is a complex activity consisting of at least several factors: the ability to differentiate and remember values and time duration rhythm, pitch (which note is higher), loudness, timbre (sound quality), and melody contour. When we sing a song or listen to some musical composition, these factors are all interwoven and we constantly make mental adjustments for them.

There is no reason to assume that all of these judgments are equally right hemisphere based, although clearly some aspects must be to produce the results already discussed. As briefly mentioned earlier, Brenda Milner tested patients with one-sided temporal lobe epilepsy before and after an operation to remove the diseased tissue. She compared their performance on tests of musical skill designed to tap just these varied aspects. She found that removal of the right temporal lobe significantly increased errors on the tests of time duration, loudness, timbre, and tonal memory (melody contour) taken from the Seashore Measures of Musical Talents.[10] These results are in fair agreement with those reporting right hemisphere dominance with normals using dichotic listening tasks. In addition, we may add that when pitch discrimination is examined, a left ear (right hemisphere) effect can be found.[11] There are some disagreements between Milner's results and the experimental attempts with normals concerning judgments of time duration and rhythm. Rhythm can be seen, of course, as a complex application of duration judgments, which Milner found to be a right dominant function. Rather than being associated with right hemisphere functioning, rhythm judgments are associated with left hemisphere superiority.

For example, Ludmil Mavlov reports a case of a musician whose stroke left him aphasic and unable to deal with rhythms, although he could imitate single tones and melodies (without rhythm). The loss of rhythmic skill was complete, whether the task was presented auditorily, visually, or through touch. In normals, it has been shown that the finer the timing distinction required to be made, the more the left hemisphere superiority seems to arise. For example, in a dichotic listening study, it was found that a right ear superiority arose when subjects had to distinguish a duration between pulses of 1/25 or 1/20 of a second, but gaps of 1/15 or 1/10 second produced no ear advantage.[12] A left hemisphere mechanism for making such fine temporal discriminations is suggestive: speech requires many, many extremely rapid discriminations. Could this be the left hemisphere basis for language? A number of researchers have suggested this is so, and the possibility will be discussed in more detail in Chapter 12. Suffice it to say for the moment that fine time discriminations may be one of the contributing factors to a left hemisphere basis for language skills.[13]

Just as not all speech sounds produce a right ear advantage equally, all tone discriminations do not produce a left ear advantage to the same extent. Pure tones, for example, are rather unreliable in producing a right hemisphere advantage. The complexity of the harmonic structure seems to be important. The more harmonic overtones embedded in the sound, the greater the left ear (right hemisphere) advantage in a dichotic listening paradigm.[14] Speech, of course, does not use steady state sounds as does music, and has no harmonic overtones as do musical instruments. So here is another possible basis for discriminating speech from music.

Emotional Factors

Notice that the nonverbal vocal sounds described earlier as producing a left ear (right hemisphere) advantage were crying, shrieking, and laughing. All are highly emotional. Recognition of them automatically involves dealing with feelings as much as with auditory perception. Similarly, one could argue that the appreciation of intonation pattern and music is highly tied to global feelings that are often very hard to express verbally. In order to truly disentangle the emotional component from perceptual ones, a number of researchers have systematically varied the emotional content of verbal material. An emotional word or phrase is no less verbal than a nonemotional one, but it may conjure up emotions as well as invoke speech recognition mechanisms. For example, emotional questions compared with nonemotional questions, tend to elicit leftward eye movements along with the response.[15] Emotion-arousing questions include: "For you, is anger or hate a stronger emotion?" and, "When you visualize your father's face, what emotion first strikes you?"

Similarly, when Robert Ley and Phil Bryden asked subjects to report the emotional expression of cartoon faces, the faces showing great joy or great anger were much better perceived in the left visual field than the right, while more neutral expressions were recognized more or less equally well on both sides.[16] More dramatic than these findings, however, are another series of experiments described in the last chapter.[17] Ley gave dichotic listening tests to subjects before and after they heard a list of words which they were to remember. The words had either positive connotations (e.g. kiss, mother, pleasure, loyalty), negative connotations (e.g. snake, morgue, greed, cancer), or were neutral (e.g. cottage, ink, apparent, bland). Also, they were either high or low in imagery, thus producing six lists. When he compared the performance on the dichotic listening tests before and after hearing the lists, he found that those trying to remember the positive and negative word lists increased their left ear (right hemisphere) score compared to those given the neutral list. High imagery word lists also increased right hemisphere performance, a point we will come back to later. Thus, it was as if the concentration on emotional words primed the right hemisphere, making it more active during the following dichotic listening task. Whether or not the right side actually increases activity (something which can only be shown with EEG measures), Ley's results do suggest a shift in dominance or lateral attention during the dichotic task.

One clear nonresult of Ley's research is the lack of a difference in lateralization changes produced by positive versus negative word lists. Some clinical researchers have claimed that positive feelings of elation or euphoria are more linked to left hemisphere functioning, while the right side is associated with negative, depressed states. The results are highly controversial and will be discussed in more detail in Chapter 14.

Visual Effects

One of the major contrasts in style of thinking involves comparing verbal thought with nonverbal, imagistic thinking. Visual ideas (or to be more accurate we should say "mental imaging" since there is no evidence that the brain's visual system is actually required) are often nonverbal in the extreme. Words are simply inadequate to describe many of these thoughts. Many psychologists claim we have at least two ways of thinking—verbal and nonverbal-visual—and that these ways constitute separate functional systems with different properties, separate rules of operation, and span of experience.[18] With such a natural division, it is easy to suggest that a hemispheric distinction corresponds to the verbal-imagery one.

Faces and Designs. Faces in general, and not just the emotional expression on them, are more easily recognized in the left visual field, indicating a right hemisphere dominance for this task. This right hemisphere dominance for face recognition has been used to explain a very dramatic effect. As Julian Jaynes describes,[19] if a line drawing face such as the upper one in Figure 6.1 is examined, fixing the gaze on the nose, the vast majority of people see it as a happy face. The lower face is seen as a sad one. Now, clearly this demonstration does not use a proper visual half field technique, since you are free to move your eyes around (see Chapter 4). Still, the effect remains. Why is this so? Jaynes suggests that because of a habitual right hemisphere dominance in facial examinations, we automatically give precedence to the side of the face on our left.

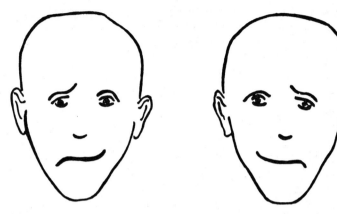

FIGURE 6.1. Most people report that the left face looks sad and that the right one looks happy. Since they are equivalent in content, the difference in judgment must be due to asymmetrical perception. Julian Jaynes (1976) suggests that this is due to right hemisphere dominance in face perception. Copyright by Julian Jaynes. Reprinted by permission.

Similarly, Morris Moscovich reports that the left side of the face of movie stars contains more expression (e.g. dimples, the winning smile, etc.) than the right side. When they show their left profile, then, these stars take advantage of this asymmetry and simultaneously put their good looks into the viewer's left visual space (given that the viewer focuses on average towards the middle of the picture).[20]

What might predispose the right hemisphere to be superior in facial recognition? Presumably it has something to do with what we look for in faces. This is cleverly demonstrated in the series of studies by Phyllis Ross and Gerald Turkewitz mentioned in Chapter 3.[21] If you recall, they presented faces for recognition in the left and right visual fields and found, not surprisingly, a range of field biases. Some subjects had a left visual field (right hemisphere) advantage and other the opposite advantage. The group with the right hemisphere bias recognized more faces correctly. Could it be that the differences between these groups is due to genuine strategy differences and not just a random variation? Their follow-up studies suggest this is so. Ross and Turkewitz altered the face stimuli in two different ways. In the first follow-up study, selective portions of the face were blocked out, such as the eyes or hairline. In the second study, the face was turned upside down. Both of these manipulations make it difficult to recognize a face, of course. Of interest here, though, is the finding that the group with the original right hemisphere bias was more affected by the second manipulation and the other group more by the first manipulation.

Thus, it appears that the left hemisphere strategy group uses an analysis of details, disrupted by blocking out specific characteristics in the face, while a right hemisphere strategy is more affected by global changes, such as inversion of the face. In normal everyday life, we recognize our friends in a global way, and may not even notice detailed changes, such as hairstyle, the loss or growth of a beard, the loss or use of glasses, and so on. Of course, our friends are usually not appreciative of the global approach when we fail to notice a change in their appearance. Yet, we could excuse ourselves by pointing out that we recognize in them and are guided by the essential qualities. Such a right hemisphere strategy may be appropriate for face recognition, but it does have its limitations.

Various types of nonfacial designs have also been tried as right hemisphere tasks. Recognition of twelve-sided nonregular polygons, for example, produces a left visual field (right hemisphere) effect.[22] However, rather than seeing which complex figures produce an asymmetry, it would be interesting to try to find what aspect of processing produces the right hemisphere bias. For example, when subjects are asked to compare the orientation of two lines or non-nameable angles (those other than verticals, horizontals, and diagonals), a left visual field advantage ensues.[23] There is also some suggestion that spatial location may be favored in the left visual field, as may perception of color.[24] The trick in getting a left visual field effect involves avoiding a verbal recoding of the stimulus. Considering the pervasiveness in our culture of verbal labelling, this is not always easy to do. One solution to controlling verbal artifacts is to present word lists, as in Ley's studies described above.

Nonverbals Skills and the Right Hemisphere

Just as language has many facets, and each facet may be independently represented in the brain, nonverbal functions are multifaceted. Here, though, there does not seem to be a concentrated conspiracy to represent all nonverbal functions in one hemisphere. Rather, we get a glimpse of the variety of factors that may distinguish the two hemispheres. Fine timing judgments seem to be dominated by left hemisphere functioning. Global visual judgments, especially of human faces, spatial judgments, and emotional judgments seem to rely more on right hemisphere activity. The language/nonlanguage distinction, so critical in our culture, may then be a misleading clue to hemisphere specialization when the details are examined.

NOTES

1. King & Kimura (1972).
2. Carmon & Nachshon (1973).
3. Kimura and Folb (1968).
4. Carmon, Lavy, Gordon & Portnoy (1975).
5. Davidson & Schwartz (1977). There are other studies reporting greater right hemisphere participation in musical tasks using different EEG paradigms. For example, Taub, Tanguay, Doubleday, Clarkson and Remington (1976) report greater evoked responses for left ear stimulation of musical chords, and Schucard, Schucard & Thomas (1977) find a greater effect on the right-sided evoked responses to unattended tone pips while subjects listen to melodies.
6. See also Smith, Chu & Edmonston (1977).
7. See Chapter 3 for a fuller discussion of split brain patients' performance.
8. Kimura (1974). Also found by Blumstein, Goodglass & Tartter (1975).
9. Blumstein & Cooper (1974).
10. Milner (1962).
11. Often no hemispheric difference is found for pitch judgments, e.g. Milner (1962) and Curry (1968), but when it is, a left ear superiority appears, as in Nachshon (1973).
12. For experimental work with normals on rhythm and duration, see Robinson & Solomon (1974), Mills & Rollman (1979), and Schwartz & Tallal (1980); the case study is found in Mavlov (1980).

13. Lackner and Teuber (1973) found left-damaged patients to be inferior to right damaged patients in perceiving separately clicks with short intervals.
14. Sidtis (1980).
15. Schwartz, Davidson and Maer (1975).
16. Ley & Bryden (1979). Similarly, when subjects have to decide whether a melody is happy or sad (determined by being in a major versus minor key), a left ear (right hemisphere) effect is found (Bryden, Ley & Sugarman, 1982).
17. Ley (1980a).
18. Paivio (1971) contrasts a verbal and an imagery system; Gazzaniga & LeDoux (1978) suggest additional systems, including motivational and emotional, each with different neurophysiological substrates.
19. Jaynes (1976). It should be noted that since a systematic test of these with different brain organization for faces, e.g. left handers (Piazza, 1980), has not been done, it is possible that the effect is due to some other factor, e.g. left to right scanning.
20. Moscovitch & Olds (1982).
21. Ross & Turkewitz (in press).
22. Dee & Fontenot (1973).
23. Umilta, Rizzolatti, Marzi, Franzini, Carmada & Berlucchi (1974).
24. Kimura (1969), but see Bryden (1976); Capitani, Scotti & Spinnler (1978).

part three

DEVELOPMENTAL ISSUES: WHEN DO (AND DID) BRAIN ASYMMETRIES APPEAR?

As with all things studied in psychology, we can ask a general developmental question about brain lateralization: How does the brain get to be lateralized? This can be interpreted in two ways, the first concerning the development within an individual person—what is the course of lateralization as the child grows? The other concerning development as a species—what is the evolutionary significance of brain lateralization?

The first question implicates the developmental issues common to developmental psychologists: Is there asymmetry at birth? Is there an increase with age? Can lateralization be affected by experiences? How does lateralization fit in with other neuropsychological aspects of the child? The second question raises issues that are more speculative because the necessary facts cannot be directly obtained. Are other animals lateralized in the same way as humans? Did Neanderthal man have an asymmetric brain? And most fundamental of all, what is the evolutionary benefit—if any—of brain lateralization?

chapter seven

Brain lateralization in the developing child

Is There an Increase in Brain Asymmetries With Age?

It had been assumed for a long time that children develop brain lateralization much as they develop adult teeth or body hair. If this were the case, the main factor of concern would be maturation, with perhaps some important environmental influences, such as the necessity for a relatively normal upbringing. In support of this view were two strong arguments, one logical and the other empirical. First of all, since the baby is born without language capabilities and language is the most obviously lateralized function, it would seem odd to consider the possibility that babies could be lateralized for something they do not have. Therefore, it was proposed, and accepted, that the child becomes lateralized slowly as he gradually develops linguistic skill. The special functions of the right hemisphere were presumed to develop also, although much less was known about the child's acquisition of visual and spatial skills.

The second argument, the empirical one, was also straightforward. In early reviews of the work done with child aphasics—

children who lose language abilities because of brain damage—two clear trends appeared: (1) children, especially young ones, generally recover their language ability, even with damage to the left hemisphere, while adults recover much more poorly; and (2) right hemisphere damage seemed as likely to produce a language loss as left hemisphere damage. Therefore, it seemed as though there was no special place in the brain for language skills until the child reached puberty.

The argument started to be questioned very soon after it was clearly articulated.[1] First, some people thought that puberty was much too late a date at which to set the beginning of lateralization. Stephen Krashen, for example, preferred five years of age, because complete recovery from aphasia is very rare after this age.[2] However, by the mid-1970s, it was clear that the arguments had to be rethought. First of all, it appeared that the chance of showing a language loss from brain damage during any period of childhood was not the same for the left and right sides. Admittedly, children with any sort of brain damage tend not to speak very much, especially to doctors in hospitals! But when more sensitive and careful measures are used for evaluating actual language loss, as opposed to reticence due to confusion, timidity, and emotional trauma, the chances are much greater that left-sided damage will produce a loss than right-sided damage.[3]

The question of children recovering language skills better than adults still had to be addressed, however, a point to which we shall return.

The logical argument given above in favor of the "lateralization by puberty" hypothesis also found a logical counterargument. Babies are constantly doing things that have no significance for them at the time, but in fact are necessary for proper development in the long term. So, although babies may not know any language, they may still be lateralized for *eventual speech*. Everything adults do has earlier forms and babies have prelinguistic skills that eventually turn into linguistic ones.[4] Perhaps these prelinguistic skills are lateralized. For example, it was shown that infants, well before they can say their first words or even understand any, can nevertheless show that they understand parts of the speech system, that they know the structure of certain basic speech sounds. Peter Eimas and his co-workers first showed that one-month-old babies distinguish the speech sounds represented by the letters *b* and *p* in the same way as adults, although in objective terms the distinction is made in an arbitrary way.[5] Other researchers have also found that very young babies seem to know a lot about speech sounds. It is as if they are born with some of this basic linguistic knowledge.[6]

No one has yet shown directly that the prelinguistic knowledge babies have is indeed lateralized. On the other hand, empirical studies on the development of lateralization for speech functions have found the same asymmetry in younger as in older children. For example, studies using dichotic listening with children of varying ages have repeatedly shown no increase in laterality with age, as shown in Figure 7.1.[7] Although older children certainly are more able to correctly detect numbers or consonant-vowel syllables they hear in the dichotic listening task than younger children, the degree to which they show a right ear advantage is not greater. Similarly, the manual tasks that have been administered to children of various ages have not shown an age trend. Thus, if there is an increase in lateralization with age, the increase must come before age two or three years, the youngest age at which the dichotic listening task has been given.

Are Young Children Lateralized in the Same Way as Older Children and Adults?

This is a difficult question to answer, because we have only indirect ways of knowing what is going on inside someone else's brain. However, young children obviously do not think like older children or adults, and have much to learn. Therefore, it very well may be that when very young children are given the dichotic listening task, they show an asymmetry for a very different reason than do older children.[8] Perhaps the younger children only think of the stimuli as sounds, while the older ones think of them as bits of words. This may mean that the youngest children are lateralized for the *perception of speech* while older children and adults are lateralized for actual *processing of language*. Since this distinction is not the sort of question one can examine directly in a two year old, we will have to wait for an answer from some ingenious experimenter.

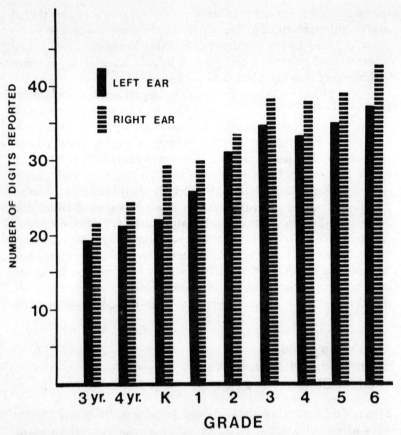

FIGURE 7.1. The advantage of the right ear over the left in processing digits in a dichotic listening task does not increase with age. From Kinsbourne & Hiscock (1977). Reproduced by permission.

Does More Lateralization
Mean Less Brain Plasticity?

It is well accepted that damage to the cortex of the brain has less of a permanent effect in young children than in older children or adults, accounting for the higher rate of recovery from aphasia in childhood. The difference is referred to by the term *brain plasticity*—the ability of the nervous system to recover a function after damage has caused the loss of it. Of course, some functions are more recoverable than others. Generally, however, the younger the child, the more likely recovery will be satisfactory. Does it not then logically follow that if young children can recover a function lost through brain damage, then that function must not have been specialized in any one spot in the brain? Not necessarily. If in fact the question of this recoverability and the question of specialization of function are independent issues, then babies can be well lateralized yet still show considerable plasticity. This simply means that we must not think of lateralization as meaning that part of the brain is "used up" or "filled" just because it is specialized for some activity.[9]

Another answer to the question of plasticity and lateralization is that we have limited ourselves by only looking at the *cortex* of the brain. Although this is considered to be the "highest" organ of the brain, the rest is also crucial and must not be ignored. Considering that the baby is born with an immature cortex, it is not too odd to think of him as a "subcortical" creature. The subcortex is very much involved in the processing of all input into the brain. The source of the lateralization may then be subcortical, and not cortical at all. How do we then account for greater brain plasticity in younger brains? One solution questions this basic assertion: Perhaps there is not such early plasticity at the level of the subcortex in the baby. It turns out that recovery of function in the baby after subcortical brain damage is considerably less likely than after cortical damage. In some ways, it is as if the locus of irretrievable specialization shifts from the subcortex to the cortex as the child grows. Also, recovery after early damage may not be as complete as we usually assume. Rather, some deficits only appear later. When the deficit does appear, it is more likely to be one of nondevelopment, rather than the loss of an acquired skill.[10]

A second solution involves finding another explanation for brain plasticity that does not rely on a lack of specialization. One way of looking at brain plasticity is to realize that the cortex changes in structure very rapidly during the first few years of life. Not only are neurons sending out connecting links to other cells (dendrites) at a prodigious rate, but there is considerable cell death as well. The high death rate (perhaps four fifths of the neurons present at birth) may be necessary for the growth of dendrites. What determines which cells will die and which will live and expand is still a mystery. However, it is easy to see how recovery of function may be a product of this growth and death process of neurons. All cortical areas are affected by input to the brain; certainly both hemispheres are. Whether one area makes more use of the information than another (i.e. whether or not there is specialization) is a separate issue, and the differential use may be due to inhibition by one area on the other areas. With brain damage to an area that is dominant for some function, other areas receiving the same input may be less inhibited now for that function and make use of the information. It may be that with a great deal of dendritic growth and selective cell death, a new area can become dominant for the function. The issue of plasticity is, however, on the frontier of brain research. We will only know whether this hypothesis is true after many more studies.

Are the Two Sides of the Brain Equipotential For Language?

Along with the general view that the children become lateralized as they get older was the view that for thinking activities, either side of the brain is *potentially* as good as the other. Clearly this does not apply completely to motor activity, such as arm and leg movements, or perceptual functions such as feeling, smelling, or seeing (see Chapter 1). But thinking functions such as speaking, doing arithmetic, or listening to music, need not be better dealt with by one side. This classical idea of *equipotentiality* was the watchword until very recently. A true test of this concept would compare the language abilities of people who have grown up from birth with only one hemisphere of the brain. In this way, we could compare the ability of the left and the right hemispheres to learn language "on their own", when brain plasticity is highest. This has been done by Maureen Dennis and her colleagues.[11] She has followed the development of children who had to have one half of their brain removed shortly after birth because of brain disease. Without such an operation the disease would have spread, and the children would have died or become very severely retarded.[12] In some of the cases, only the cortex had to be surgically removed from one side. Instead of being severely retarded, these children had a weakening of motor control on the side opposite to the side of brain damage (a *hemiparesis*), but had normal IQ scores. To the casual observer, there seems to be no difference between the children with only a left or only a right functioning brain, other than which side is paralyzed. However, upon closer examination with sensitive tests of language abilities, it turns out that the isolated left hemisphere is better at grammatical skills, while the isolated right hemisphere is better at some perceptual skills. Although the children with only a right hemisphere could read satisfactorily, they seemed to function without much aid of phonics.[13]

Is There Any Evidence of Asymmetry At Birth?

It seems logical that if in fact babies are born with some linguistic or prelinguistic knowledge, perhaps this knowledge is lateralized to one side of the brain. This is in fact now assumed to be the case, although as mentioned before, it is far from clear whether the left hemisphere bias for speech in infants exists for the same reasons as it does for adults. The first report of such a left bias for speech was by Dennis Molfese.[14] He measured EEGs from newborn babies and played a tape recording of speech sounds (consonant-vowel syllables) and musical sounds (piano chords). Using the method of averaged evoked responses (as described in Chapter 4), he found that the left hemisphere generally gave a larger response to the speech sounds than the right hemisphere did. The opposite was the case with the musical sounds.

Shortly after this report, Anne Kasman Entus announced a similar finding using a combination of the dichotic listening procedure and a habituation paradigm, called HAS for *high amplitude sucking*.[15] In this ingenious setup, the baby sucks on a pacifier that is hooked up to a pressure transducer and tape recorder. When the baby sucks above a certain rate, the stimulus is played. As long as he continues sucking, he keeps hearing the stimulus. So, if the baby gets bored with what he is hearing, he can do something about it. In this way, Entus could see whether 2½-month-old babies can perceive interesting changes in one ear better than the other, as shown in Figure 7.2. She played tapes of speech or of musical instruments, and

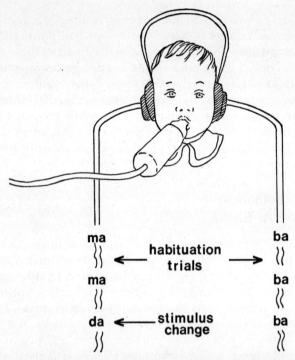

FIGURE 7.2. The HAS paradigm merged with dichotic listening allows the baby to control the input. Entus (1977) reports that the babies responded more to an opportunity to listen to a change in speech sound in the right ear and music in the left ear. The picture depicts the right-ear-change-with-speech condition.

found that with right ear stimulation, the babies tended to show more of a response to new speech sounds, while with left ear input, there was more response to new musical sounds. Thus, once again it seems that babies do not treat speech and musical stimuli symmetrically.

Other studies have pushed the earliest age of lateralization for speech back to before full gestation by testing the reactions of premature babies to speech and music,[16] and expanded considerably the measures used.[17] Most studies with newborn babies have looked for left hemisphere specialization—that is, for hemisphere specialization for some language-related task. However, Barerra and her colleagues found evidence for right hemisphere specialization too.

Babies looked more to their left to see a picture of mother than to the right, an indication that the right hemisphere seems to be more involved in this task.

These studies all concerned asymmetries in psychological functioning. By this we mean that the brain seems to process the stimulation in an asymmetric way. The stimulation must, then, mean something to the babies, even if only that they know the difference between it and other stimulation. To some extent, this means that the brain is preprogrammed to recognize what speech will sound like, compared to music for example. Obviously, babies do not know the meanings of words, but to some extent, the newborn does not have an entirely naive brain. One conclusion from this is that, in some sense, babies are born with some knowledge of the nature of speech sounds.

When Does Handedness Start?

We can also ask about brain asymmetries not related to psychological functioning, for example *handedness*. How soon do right-handed people become right-handed? How soon do left-handed people show evidence of being left-handed? To study this, we could examine a large number of babies at birth or shortly after birth. We could also follow up a few babies from birth into childhood when handedness will be well established. This second approach is very expensive in time and money, but one such longitudinal study was done by Arnold Gesell and Louise Ames in the 1930s and 1940s.[18] They took movies of babies periodically until they had grown up into 10 year old children. From a painstaking analysis of the resulting films, they found that hand preference switched a number of times in the first year of life, and settled clearly by about two years of age.

This kind of study requires heroic patience and foresight. A much more convenient method involves testing a larger number of babies just once or only a few times. The advantages are obvious: Results are obtained faster and so it is easier to follow up the study with more research. Imagine conducting a ten-year study and then discovering that a different task should have been given at the start! It is not surprising that a number of short-term infant handedness studies have been done.

Although we have an intuitive idea of what handedness means to us as adults, it is less clear for infants. (A more complete discussion is given in Chapter 9.) Should we look at how strong each hand is? Which hand will hold onto an object longer? Which hand is used for reaching objects? A number of such measures have been used with variable results. When differences between the hands have been found, they are found at a much earlier age than Gesell and Ames' study. For example, babies within the first six months of life show a tendency to grasp more with the right hand and cling more with the left hand.[19] On the other hand, the right hand has been found to hold onto a rattle longer in a group of 16-week-olds and this has been replicated a number of times at even younger ages.[20] Similarly, the strength of the grasp reflex of the right hand is stronger than that of the left hand in babies as young as three weeks.[21] These results were all found in a group of babies whose parents are all right-handed, and who we would expect will also turn out to be right-handed.

There is evidence, however, to favor a "left-then-right" handedness theory. For example, there is a left hand preference for reaching for and manipulating objects. This left bias gradually shifts to a right bias over a number of weeks, the preference change depending to some extent on the object to be manipulated. For example, the left hand preference lasts until 28 weeks of age for a cube, 32 weeks for a pellet, and even as late as 44 to 52 weeks for a bell.[22]

The differences between hand preference in infants, when found, are not large, and it may be useful to examine the two hands in natural settings. Instead of comparing which one does *more* of something, we could look to see whether they naturally do *different* things. For example, Francois Bresson and his colleagues did a detailed analysis of hand movements of babies from 17 to 40 weeks of age while reaching for objects. They concluded that the two hands play complementary roles, the left devoted to one sort of localizing function and the right is devoted to another localizing function and to handling.[23] If both hands have their own special roles, the seemingly contradictory results mentioned earlier are no longer confusing. The left *is* preferred for some activities, the right for most others. As Bresson points out, there are a number of skills the left hand is better at even in right-handed adults and children, all related to the right hemisphere superiority in spatial tasks.[24]

There are other bodily asymmetries besides those involving hands. For example, people generally prefer to use one eye more than the other when sighting in a telescope, microscope, or keyhole. This preference is quite independent of visual acuity of each eye. Rather, it is akin to "handling" something visually. Similarly, people are consistent with an ear preference, as shown by asking someone to listen to a conversation through a keyhole. Of course, there is also a foot preference, for kicking a ball, for example. The correlations between these preferences is amazingly low. Although hand and foot preference go together somewhat, neither go together with eye and ear preference. So, there are many right-handed, right-footed individuals who have a left eye or left ear preference.[25]

Obviously, our culture is biased in favor of right hand use, but it is hard to imagine how one could pressure someone to prefer one eye or ear over the other. Indeed, the frequency of right bias is much lower for the ear (1.3 to 1) and eye (2.2 to 1) than for the foot (4 to 1) and hand (6.7 to 1). Consistent with this cultural effect is the finding that the right preference for hand and foot increases continuously through life while ear and eye preferences do not show such a trend, as seen in Figure 7.3.

The fact, however, that there is an asymmetric bias for eye and ear preferences indicates that much more than cultural influences are involved. There must be some biological basis to the asymmetry, although it may not be total.

Can Brain Lateralization Be Affected During the Child's Growth by Experience?

This question raises the heredity-environment debate once again. Although we now know that the child is born with definite brain asymmetries and possibly some long term predispositions, we do not know to what extent, if any, lateralization can be molded.

It is perhaps easier to deal with handedness first. Although school teachers and parents tried for many generations to force children who preferred to write with their left hands to switch to their right, the result was often very unsatisfactory. Often the children ended up using their left anyway or ended up frustrated. Of course,

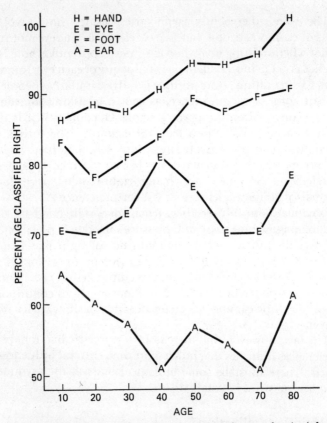

FIGURE 7.3. The relative incidence of a preference for the left versus right side differs for various parts of the body, although changes are relatively small over the life-span. From Porac, Coren & Duncan (1980). Reprinted by permission.

some people are genuinely ambidextrous, and write with one hand and throw a ball with the other.

The issue of nature (heredity) versus nurture (environment) in brain asymmetries for psychological functions is not at all clear. Although it is tempting to think of brain lateralization as an immutable biological function, we must also remember that the brain is the organ of the mind. Just as the structure of the mind may change through experience, so might the organization of the mind in the brain change. From what we have discussed so far, it is clear that there are predispositions, for example, for the left hemisphere to be more involved in speech processing. But can significant experiences change the ultimate outcome?

Some professions tend to involve styles of thinking different from others. For example, lawyers engage in left hemisphere-type tasks more often than artists, whose activities seem to be based in the right hemisphere. Does this mean lawyers and artists have different brain lateralization, either previous to choosing their professions or as a result of them? This issue is discussed in detail in Chapter 11.

By way of summary, however, we find that the issue of brain organization may be separate from the issue of capability. That is, when an individual does have a skill, it is most likely to be organized in his brain in a standard way, despite the degree of excellence (or lack thereof) in the skill. There are those who disagree with this, though, and claim that a person's mental skills do affect his brain organization. For example, Ralph Cameron reported that right brain-damaged patients are much more likely to lose language skills if they were illiterate before their accident.[26] It appears that literacy may encourage left lateralization for language. Perhaps schooling teaches youngsters to think of language in an analytic way, a style of thinking associated with left hemisphere function.

Similarly, some claim that learning a second language affects brain organization, and that the age at which the second language is learned is critical. Although their arguments are still considered speculative, it would be surprising if bilingualism had no effect on brain organization.[27]

There is a very difficult problem, however, in this question. Brain lateralization is measured by administering certain tasks. No matter what measure we use, we are really measuring the results of behavior based on those tasks. If we find a difference in asymmetry between two groups, is it because the groups choose to solve the task differently? How can we be sure that any two people are doing the same thing mentally? When illiterates seem to be less left-lateralized for language than literates, it may be that they perceive and treat the task of communication differently from schooled literates. If language is something different to them, it is not surprising that it should be organized differently. Similarly, as was discussed in Chapter 5, since in Japan reading is not an entirely analytic, phono-logically based task, Japanese aphasics do not have the same difficulty with reading as English-speaking aphasics. Similarly, as discussed earlier, when subjects hear a sound in a speech context, they show a left hemisphere bias, but when the same sound is presented with music the bias switches.[28]

We are left, then, with the conclusion that there is little evidence that a specific early experience can alter lateralization for a specific mental function. This does not mean, however, that the early experience won't change the individual's preferred way of thinking or his attitude toward specific tasks.

Is Anatomy Destiny?

To what extent are the asymmetries in brain functioning related to anatomical asymmetries? As we discussed in Chapter 1, the two halves of the brain are never exactly the same (just as the two sides of one's face are different). However, these differences are not random: some of the language processing area in the left temporal lobe is generally larger than the homologous area on the right even in neonatal and fetal brains.[29] Does this mean that hemispheric differences are set at birth?

This is a very difficult question to answer because for an individual, we can never know the degree of asymmetry until after death. Clearly the brains of neonates cannot be examined and then the individuals followed through life. The only solution is to test people thoroughly on neuropsychological tests and then examine their brains after death. When results like these are in, we will be in a better position to answer this question.

We have dealt with a number of intriguing questions in this chapter, including many for which we will have to wait for answers. One can see all the issues of how the mind and brain are related being amplified in the developmental perspective. Yet it is here that the most basic questions will be answered: To what extent does the baby come into the world with a lateralized brain? How is it lateralized in adulthood? And how does it get from here to there?

We now have good reason to believe that some asymmetries in cerebral organization exist at birth, at least for the processing of speech sounds and maybe also for visual-spatial stimuli. Clearly there seem to be more hemisphere differences in adults than these, and we cannot be sure how they come about. It could be that there are really no changes in lateralization. Rather, the new activities the child learns as he grows up make use of speech or visual-spatial processes and are lateralized to the extent that they use them. It could also be that some complex activity, such as the sequencing of sounds necessary to form words, becomes lateralized because of its usual association with an already lateralized function, such as speech. A third possibility is that everything that is lateralized in adults is already lateralized at birth, but it is hard to figure out how to test these functions in infants. These possibilities all have evidence in favor of them and may all be correct to some degree.[30]

NOTES

1. For example, by Lenneberg (1967, Chapter 4).
2. Krashen (1973).
3. Kinsbourne & Hiscock (1977).
4. See Bower (1977) for a readable and delightful discussion of the intellectual capacities of newborn babies.
5. Eimas, Siqueland, Juscyk & Vigorito (1971). The method they used is the high amplitude sucking technique described below.
6. See Trehub (1979) and Molfese & Molfese (1979b) for recent reviews.
7. Good demonstrations of the constancy of the effect throughout childhood are reported by Berlin, Hughes, Lowe-Bell & Berlin (1973), Piazza (1977) and Hiscock & Kinsbourne (1977,1980). For an extensive review see Witelson (1977d).
8. Porter & Berlin (1975).
9. See Moscovitch (1977) for a discussion of this. For discussion on the nature of brain plasticity, see Stein, Rosen & Butters (1974) and Huttenlocher (1979), but see St. James-Roberts (1981) for alternative explanations of evidence for plasticity.
10. Kohn & Dennis (1974b).
11. Kohn & Dennis (1974a); Dennis & Whitaker (1976, 1977); Dennis (1979).
12. Hoffman, Hendrick, Dennis & Armstrong (1979).
13. Dennis, Lovett & Weigel-Crump (1981).

14. Molfese, Freeman & Palermo (1975).
15. Entus (1977). There is currently some doubt cast on whether this method is reliable. Vargha-Khadem & Corballis (1979) tried to repeat Entus' findings and failed. However, they did make a small change in the procedure of the testing, replacing the human experimenter who inserted the pacifier into the baby's mouth with a mechanical arm. Whether or not these results stand remains to be seen. What is clear, though, is that lateralization is not always easy to detect!
16. Segalowitz & Chapman (1980).
17. Glanville, Best & Levenson (1977), Gardiner & Walter (1977), Molfese & Molfese (1979a) and Barerra, Dalrymple & Witelson (1978). See Segalowitz (mimeo) for a review.
18. Gesell & Ames (1947).
19. Halverson (1937 a,b).
20. Caplan & Kinsbourne (1976), Petrie & Peters (1979).
21. Peters & Petrie (1979).
22. Seth (1973). See Young (1977) for an excellent review and Young, Corter, Segalowitz & Trehub (in press) for further studies on this topic.
23. Bresson, Maury, Pierant-Le Bonniec & de Schonen (1977).
24. Hermelin & O'Conner (1971), Ingram (1975).
25. Coren, Porac & Duncan (1981).
26. Cameron, Currier & Haerer (1971).
27. Albert & Obler (1978); Vaid & Genesee (1981); compare Paradis (1977).
28. Spellacy & Blumstein (1970).
29. Witelson & Pallie (1973); Wada, Clarke & Hamm (1975).
30. See Segalowitz (mimeo) for a review of the infant lateralization research and discussion of these three models.

chapter eight

The evolution of lateralization

Is brain lateralization unique to humans? There are, of course, many psychological and neurological factors that differentiate us from other animals. We may reasonably ask whether an asymmetrical brain is one of them. If so, then perhaps lateralization is a property that underlies some of the unique aspects of the human mind. For example, among the cognitive skills that have been suggested as separating the human mind from all others are language capabilities and consciousness. It is conceivable that brain lateralization as a biological function is related in some important way to these human dimensions. If, on the other hand, we find good evidence for cerebral dominance in lower animals, lateralization is probably more related to simple perceptual functions. Before we speculate on the grander implications of the development of lateralization in human evolution, let us examine the evidence for asymmetries in non-humans, and discover wherein which level of the brain's structure these capacities lie.

EVIDENCE FOR BRAIN LATERALIZATION IN ANIMALS

Neuroanatomical Data

The upper surface of the left temporal lobe in humans, specifically the planum temporale, which is intimately involved in language processing, is generally larger in the left hemisphere than in the right. Although no one has demonstrated explicitly that asymmetry of size is related to the well-known asymmetry of functions, it is certainly tempting to suggest that this is more than just a coincidence. Are physical brain asymmetries found in other animals? Some have been found in our closest phylogenetic relatives, nonhuman primates. The planum temporale is not so easily measured in nonhumans because the folds in the nonhuman brain do not make it so distinct. However, other less direct measurements have proved useful, most notably the height and length of the Sylvian fissure (see Figure 8.1). In humans, the Sylvian fissure generally rises to a higher point on the right side.

Marjorie LeMay and Norman Geschwind examined a number of brains of Old and New World monkeys, other lesser apes, and great

FIGURE 8.1. The Sylvian fissure, which demarcates the upper border of the temporal lobe, is usually higher in the right hemisphere, contributing to the anatomical asymmetries found in the language zones. See Rubens (1977) for more detail.

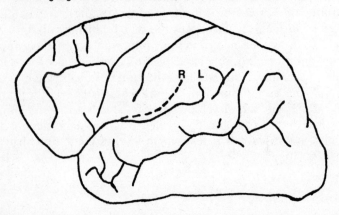

TABLE 8.1. Comparison of human and nonhuman primate neuroanatomical asymmetries.

	ANIMAL	NUMBER EXAMINED	L > R	L = R	R > L
Height of Sylvian Fissure					
LeMay & Culebras (1972)	humans	44	2 (5%)	4 (9%)	38 (86%)
Hochberg & LeMay (1975)	humans	106	7 (7%)	28 (26%)	71 (67%)
LeMay & Geschwind (1975)	monkeys and lesser apes	41	0	38 (93%)	3 (7%)
	great apes:				
	total	28	1 (4%)	11 (39%)	16 (57%)
	orangutan	12	0	2 (17%)	10 (83%)
	chimpanzee	9	1 (11%)	4 (44%)	4 (44%)
	gorilla	7	0	5 (71%)	2 (29%)
Length of Sylvian fissure					
Yeni-Komshian & Benson (1976)	humans	25	21 (84%)	0	4 (16%)
	chimpanzees	25	20 (80%)	3 (12%)	2 (8%)
	Rhesus monkeys	25	11 (44%)	9 (36%)	5 (20%)
Fischer (1921, as quoted in Witelson, 1977b)	chimpanzees	24	12 (50%)	8 (33%)	4 (17%)

apes. It should be kept in mind that in terms of evolutionary history, humans are much closer relatives of great apes than of the other primates. Lemay and Geschwind found asymmetries in only 3 of 41 monkeys and lesser apes, while of 28 great apes, there were 16 with the right side higher and only 1 with the left side larger (see Table 8.1). This asymmetry tends to produce a longer Sylvian fissure on the left side with a longer planum temporale, since this structure is part of the surface of the fissure. Similarly, a longer left-sided Sylvian fissue is found in humans and in chimpanzees, but not in rhesus monkeys.

Thus, our close phylogenetic relationship to the great apes is reflected in at least one asymmetry in brain structure.[1]

Other neuroanatomical asymmetries exist in humans besides those involving language areas. If brain asymmetries correspond to functional asymmetries, it may be that others are more likely to be found in nonhuman primates than are the language related ones because only humans have natural language. However, these other areas are less well-explored.[2]

What is the evolutionary significance of the anatomical asymmetries found in nonhuman primates? Let us assume for a moment that the greater planum temporale in the left hemisphere does have something to do with language functions. Other animals do not have the language abilities of adult humans, despite the recent successes at teaching hand signs to some of the great apes.[3] The evolutionary process does not promote the development of structures for *future* use, but only for present advantage. Therefore some perceptual or cognitive functions, whether they are very simple or highly complex, must benefit from the asymmetries, presumably by itself being asymmetrically represented in the brain. Unfortunately, the evidence for such functional asymmetries in nonhumans, to which we now turn, is not overwhelming.

Are There Functional Asymmetries in Nonhumans?

Being species-centric, we might expect that the most positive reports of lateralization among nonhumans could be among primates, our nearest relatives. So let us begin with them.

Nonhuman Primates. Attempts to find lateralization effects in monkeys use tasks analogous to those with humans involving vision.[4] Of course, it is not easy to be sure that the animals are using the same perceptual processes as people when responding to the tasks; nevertheless, whereas humans show definite asymmetries with color, shape, and orientation tasks, monkeys do not. Similarly, facial recognition and shape discrimination failed to produce the asymmetry found in humans (favoring the right hemisphere). No asymmetry was found with split-brain monkeys on a visual sequencing task.[5]

Researchers have been more successful with auditory tasks. On an auditory discrimination task, a deficit was found in four out of four left hemisphere damage cases, while neither of the two right hemishpere damaged monkeys were deficient in the task.[6]

More suggestive than this was a variation of the dichotic listening task used with monkeys. Japanese macaques and other Old World monkeys listened to vocalizations of Japanese macaques in only one ear on each trial. They were expected to indicate an ability to distinguish two natural vocalizations—one produced mainly by estrous females soliciting male consorts, the other a more general social signal produced by all of the monkeys—by releasing a gripped bar when one but not the other of the sounds was heard. They received a food reinforcement for the correct response. All of the monkeys could do the task well, but all five of the Japanese macaques did significantly better when the vocalization was presented to the right ear, implying that the left hemisphere is superior in making the judgment. Only one of the five non-Japanese macaque control monkeys showed a similar right ear advantage. Thus, speech sounds that mean something to the monkeys are better processed in the left hemisphere. The parallel with human speech lateralization on the dichotic listening task is striking.

Lower Animals. It could very well be that hemispheric functional asymmetries exist in many species of animals, but that we do not know what to look for. Our main distinction for humans is the verbal-nonverbal dichotomy, but for other animals this is usually an irrelevant dimension. We have seen that in Japanese macaque monkeys, vocalization is a relevant variable. This is also the case with some varieties of birds. Fernando Nottebohm discovered that canaries and chaffinches have left-sided control of their bird song. He did this by noting the effects of severing the left or the right hypoglossal nerve.[7]

As we have seen, many functions are asymmetrically represented besides those dealing with speech. All mammals seem to experience levels of emotionality and to have characteristic ways of showing it, whether or not they have complex communication systems. For example, rats clearly do not have speech, but emotionality can easily be noted by measuring activity level. When rats are very excited they tend to "freeze" on the spot rather than explore their surroundings. Emotionality in rats has been linked to asymmetrical brain function. Victor Denenberg and his colleagues found that for rats with a somewhat stimulating rearing, removal of the left cerebral cortex only changes the level of emotionality minimally. Right-sided decortication, however, vastly affected the exploration behavior.[8]

In another study, the activity level of rats was examined after left versus right brain damage caused by stopping the blood flow in the main artery. The activity level of the left-damaged animals, as measured by the number of revolutions in a running wheel, stayed the same after they recovered from the operation. The right-damaged group, however, became quite hyperactive.[9]

This evidence suggests a lateralized representation of some emotional function. Clearly the results are not completely similar to those in humans, but then again, rats are not people. What is important is the finding that some *psychological* function may be lateralized in some lower animals. These studies are, however, meager help for the otherwise bleak prospects of detecting lateralization in animals. The study of paw preference does not brighten those prospects.

Paw Preference. One of the undeniable asymmetries in humans is the overwhelming preference for the right hand in tasks requiring agility. Although hand preference is not tied directly to the pattern of lateralization, the bias is very large and suggestive of something asymmetric in the brain. Can similar consistent handedness be found so clearly in animals? The answer, in a word, is no. Although there is the occasional intriguing report of a consistent preference in a species—for example, all eight gorillas studied led off their chest beating with the right arm[10]—it is more usual to find individual preferences only. A particular animal may prefer one paw over the other, but in a large group the number of left and right preferences are likely to be equal. Within an individual animal, there may be a right paw preference for some tasks and a left for other tasks. There can even be changes of paw preference over time.[11] Clearly, humans differ from other animals rather drastically in their consistency of preference and in their bias toward the right.

WHAT IS THE EVOLUTIONARY
ADVANTAGE OF LATERALIZATION?

Despite whatever advantages we may postulate for cerebral asymmetries in humans today, we must find some evolutionary advantage if we are to account for them. Such benefits may be intellectual, in terms of perceptual skills, memory processes, or linguistic abilities, or may involve improved motor skills. Attempts to develop evolutionary accounts are hampered, of course, by the dearth of information concerning lateralization elsewhere in the animal kingdom. There are many, many documented anatomical asymmetries in all sorts of animals, including such arcane tidbits as that in birds, the left ovary is larger than the right and the existence of the left one inhibits the growth of the other.[12] However, cerebral asymmetries for higher functions, whether they be motor coordination, spatial representation of the world, or linguistic-symbolic coding, are not plentiful outside of humans in the animal kingdom, as we have seen. The ones we have mentioned—occasional findings ranging from songbirds' representation of bird song to various neuroanatomical asymmetries in great apes to species-specific cries in Japanese macaques—do not lend themselves to an orderly reconstruction of phylogenetic development! Therefore the theories are definitely of a speculative nature.

Are There Cognitive Benefits
to Lateralization?

Crowded Brains and Poor Performance. Jerre Levy has suggested that there is a functional benefit to keeping different thinking skills separate in the brain. If verbal-analytic thinking is really different from (and is even incompatible with) spatial-holistic thinking, then a brain that mixes the neuropsychological functions involved in them will have a handicap. It should be easier and more efficient to keep the processes as separate as possible.

Levy argues that this principle would only apply to an organism that depends a great deal on abstract thought, that is, humans and perhaps other "higher" animals. Nonabstract thought

131

is tied to the external world, which is not laterally biased. Therefore, there would be no particular benefit for lower organisms to be lateralized. As Levy says,

> A bilaterally symmetrical brain, while serving quite well to map a bilaterally symmetrical body and an unbiased external space, is an enormously wasteful design for a neural computer whose primary and most important function is the construction of models of reality and plans for behavior that encompass the evolutionary and individual past and imagine the future.[13]

She predicts that those who are bilateralized for language should be lower in spatial skills, since language skills "crowd out" or interfere with the nonverbal talents (this assumes, of course, that language skills predominate).[14] Left-handers are a group with less left-lateralization for language generally (discussed further in the next chapter), so we should expect to find lower spatial skills in left-handers if this theory is correct. Although Levy did report such results on a small group, generally such differences are not found. With a representative sample of 7,119 children between the ages of 6 and 11 years, no differences in verbal or nonverbal skills were found between left and right handers.[15] Less laterality does not seem to be a cognitive liability.

Handedness and Babbling. Marcel Kinsbourne suggests a different route for the eventual functional asymmetry of speech (nonverbal skills are not discussed in this model).[16] First, he suggests it is symmetry that must be explained, not asymmetry. He says it is advantageous to have equal hand dexterity since this promotes quick, accurate action, such as in hunting. Once food is retrieved, however, the adaptive pressure for symmetry is relieved and hand or paw specialization becomes reasonable and even preferable. Let us accept that, for whatever reason, the right hand becomes the preferred one, so that for skilled movements the left hemisphere predominates. Speech is a highly complicated motor function and thus would naturally be served by the left hemisphere, and there would be no adaptive pressure for it to be bilaterally represented. Also, Kinsbourne suggests that the pointing a child does while babbling as it learns to speak reinforces this left hemisphere basis.[17]

This model is based on a number of assumptions—that asymmetry is the norm unless there is some pressure to be symmetrical, that there is an inherited predisposition to be right-handed in most people, and that hemisphere specialization for motor functions controls both hand preference and side of speech dominance. No one has yet demonstrated whether symmetry or asymmetry is the norm, although many arguments can be made concerning this.[18] The second assumption—that right hand preference is inherited—seems obviously true, and yet the data are still lacking (see Chapter 9). The third implies that *all* right-handers should be left dominant for speech and that all left handers should be right dominant for speech. This is clearly not the case, although it may be that exceptions can be accounted for by birth trauma to some degree. This hypothesis is explored further in the next chapter.

Reduction of Conflict Through Specialization. Consistent with Levy's "crowding" hypothesis is the notion that it is advantageous for abstract thinking to be localized in one hemisphere. In other words, two somewhat separate half-brains (not split-brains) can be more efficient than one completely integrated one. Joseph Bogen, one of the pioneers in the split-brain research, reasons this way too. With two hemispheric styles that are considerably distinct, there is a greater probability of finding solutions to problems—presuming that there are not two conflicting solutions, each favored by a different hemisphere![19]

Specialization may also help reduce interhemispheric conflict. When a motor command is given, one hemisphere is dominant for that instruction, for example, the right hemisphere for left leg movements. If both hemispheres undertake abstract decisions, with neither being dominant, however, there is the possibility of conflict. Dominance, that is, asymmetry of decision-making for some particular task, would reduce such conflict should it arise.[20]

As we saw in Chapter 4, there is some evidence that conflict between actions is reduced if they are grounded in separate hemispheres rather than in the same hemisphere. These results could be considered support for the "conflict" hypothesis. Unfortunately, counterevidence can be found in the same place as that for the "crowding" hypothesis. Less lateralized people should be less efficient, and this has not been shown to be the case.

What is the Evolutionary Advantage of Handedness?

There must be some general benefit to being "handed", that is, to having a general preference for using one hand over the other. We can easily accept that it is better to stick to one hand for routine activities that require practice. Training both hands can take twice as long as training one only, as any musician knows when trying to play an instrument with hands reversed. Not only must the muscles conform to the requirements of the activity, but so too must the mental planning needed. This planning does not entirely generalize across hemispheres, and so it makes sense that the hands should specialize. This is what we see in animals. A general predisposition to use one hand would capitalize on any transfer of skill from one activity to another.

This would not mean that the unpreferred hand should be ignored. Rather, the hypothesis just outlined would argue for a *complementary* use of each hand, where the two learn to cooperate by a division of labor. The preferred hand does anything that requires agility and fine movements, while the other makes the situation ready, such as by holding or steadying the object to be acted on.[21]

Why the Right Hand? The choice of the right hand as the preferred one most of the time in humans may have been an historical accident that was reinforced by culture. It is more likely, though, that the choice has biological significance, because if the choice of side of preference is arbitrary, we should expect to find some cultures with a left bias. No such cultures have ever been found.[22]

What sort of biological pressure could predispose people to prefer the right hand? Michael Corballis and his colleagues propose that there is a gradient of development in the body of all animals, that favors the *left* side of the body and the brain. Since it is the left hemisphere that controls the fine coordination of the right hand, people tend to be right-handed.[23] There is no definitive empirical support for this hypothesis, although it is theoretically attractive, since then the "advanced" hemisphere would take care of the most "advanced" intellectual function—language. However, one could argue for the opposite hypothesis and come up with the same result. Several sets of researchers working on the blood flow patterns in the brain have found that right-handers have a greater blood flow on the *right* side of the brain.[24] Let us infer from this that the right side is more maturationally advanced. The first complex activities of the newborn infant involve visual-spatial reckoning. Perhaps this is why these skills are right-lateralized. The later developing functions of speech and manual agility may be subsumed by the remaining hemisphere. This hypothesis, which is the reverse of Corballis's, is clearly grossly speculative. Perhaps it is best an illustration of the extent to which we are driven to guesswork by our lack of facts.[25]

What is Adaptive About Left-Handedness? If right-handedness was such a success evolutionarily, some benefit must be found for left hand preference, since its existence has been relatively constant over the millenia.[26] Certainly, left-handers have been discriminated against in the modern world. Common items from telephone booths to can openers to scissors are designed in favor of right-handers.[27] Historically, however, we must assume that some benefit accrues to being different in this way. Two possibilities include "battle fitness" and "accident" fitness. As any right-hander knows who plays tennis against a left-handed opponent, the surprise factor and the change in tactics required benefit the left-hander. Presumably this was so prehistorically as well and may have outweighed any social isolation due to the eccentricity. The advantage only occurs, of course, as long as left-handers remain a minority. As well, left-handers tend to recover better from localized brain damage, which is clearly a survival advantage, although not necessarily a reproductive advantage.

However, since we do not know for sure what it is that causes hand preference, it may be that left-handedness is an incidental by-product of some altogether unknown factor for which there are strong adaptive pressures.

Which Came First, Handedness or Cognitive Lateralization?

To some extent, this is a chicken-or-egg question, although it is also conceivable that each has nothing to do with the origin of the other. For example, it is possible that human linguistic skills have developed (evolutionarily) from gestural systems.[28] People do gesture more with the right hand while speaking, while other hand movements, such as self-touching, are not right-biased.[29] Thus, one could argue that linguistic skills are left-lateralized because they are evolutionarily based on gestural communication in which the right hand plays a leading role since it is more agile.

If the above theory is the chicken's side of the story, let us also examine the egg's perspective. We know that nonhuman primates and other animals are quite capable of hand preference, but that consistent preference within the species is not found. We also know that some primates are capable of at least primitive sign language and that sign language does not especially favor one hand over the other. So it is entirely conceivable from present evidence that the cognitive prerequisites for linguistic communication precede consistent handedness in primates. The advantage homo sapiens acquired was a vocal tract, tongue, and mouth cavity that made verbal communication flexible and convenient.[30] The new-found linguistic skills, however, required great motor coordination of the tongue, lips, vocal tract, and breathing. As was argued earlier, there is benefit to having one hemisphere control complex motor programming, and whichever hemisphere was given this task may become preeminent for motor coordination tasks in general.[31] Certainly this is the case. The left hemisphere shows a clear superiority in timing and sequencing tasks and coordination in motor planning. Therefore, the (almost) consistent right hand preference in humans could be due to the appearance of lateralization for a cognitive function rather than the other way around. This theory, like the others, does not account for the persistent problem of left handers, for their lateralization pattern is not simply reversed.

NOTES

1. LeMay & Geschwind (1975); Yeni-Komshian & Benson (1976); see Witelson (1977b) and Galaburda, LeMay, Kemper & Geschwind (1978) for summaries of this work.
2. Cain & Wada (1979) report 6 of 7 baboon brains they examined have a longer frontal lobe on the right, as is found with humans.

3. See Linden (1974) for a summary of this research. However, as Pettito & Seidenberg (1979) and Terrace (1979) point out, there is more to human language use than knowledge of signs. Thus, whether the signing capabilities recently discovered in chimpanzees and gorillas constitutes linguistic skill on a human scale is still an open question.
4. See Hamilton (1977) for a review.
5. Warren & Nonneman (1976).
6. Dewson (1977).
7. Nottebohm (1979). This research arises again in the Chapter 10 in the discussion on sex differences.
8. Denenberg, Garbanati, Sherman, Yutzey & Kaplan (1978). These results involve complex interactions with the degree of stimulation in early experiences, which we need not explore here.
9. Robinson (1979).
10. Schaller (1963).
11. See Warren (1977) and Hamilton (1977) for reviews.
12. Warren (1977), Morgan & Corballis (1978).
13. Levy (1977).
14. Levy (1969).
15. Roberts & Engle (1974, cited in Kinsbourne, 1978). Similar non-differences are reported by Newcombe & Ratcliffe (1973) and are reviewed extensively by Hardyck, Petrinovich & Goldman (1976).
16. Kinsbourne (1978).
17. Kinsbourne & Lempert (1979).
18. See Kinsbourne (1978); also Corballis & Morgan (1978) and Morgan & Corballis (1978).
19. Bogen & Bogen (1969).
20. Corballis & Beale (1976, pp. 98–99).
21. This is essentially the pattern that is found as the infant develops this complementarity between the hands, as discussed by Bresson, Maury, Pierant-Le Bonniec & deSchonen (1977).
22. Coren & Porac (1977).
23. Corballis & Beale (1976); Corballis & Morgan (1978); Morgan & Corballis (1978).
24. Carmon & Gombos (1970) and, more recently, Prohovnik, Hakansson & Risberg (1980) found greater right-sided blood

flow in right handers and greater left-sided flow in left handers.

25. Or too many facts! See Segalowitz & Gruber (1977c) for a summary of four possible explanations for the pattern of lateralization. I should point out that none accounts for the different lateralization patterns in left handers.

26. See Harris (1980) and Corballis & Beale (1976) for historical summaries. Bakan (1971, 1977) has offered an alternative proposal: that left handedness is not an adaptation, but rather an accident everywhere it is found. He suggests all left handers have mild brain damage due to anoxia at birth. This argument is treated further in the following chapter.

27. See Barsley (1970) for more on the world of the left hander.

28. See Harnad, Steklis & Lancaster (1976).

29. Kimura (1973).

30. Lieberman (1975).

31. Kimura & Archibald (1974).

part four

INDIVIDUAL DIFFERENCES: HOW (AND WHY) ARE PEOPLE DIFFERENT?

So far we have covered the typically accepted characteristics of the left and right hemispheres and reviewed much of the evidence for these asymmetries. We have treated everyone as having the same pattern of brain asymmetries, as if all left hemispheres and all right hemispheres were alike. However, as in everything else in life, there are differences from person to person. We can ask whether these differences are systematic enough so that we may group individuals together by their patterns of brain asymmetries. If we can account for individual differences in lateralization by means of other factors, such as hand preference or choice of vocation, we will have gone a long way toward understanding the organization of the brain. Conversely, if we find that people who are different in terms of personality or intellectual factors are also different in specific patterns of brain organization, we may understand more deeply what it is that makes for such personality and intellectual differences.

There are basically three ways for individuals to be different in brain lateralization.

1. The brain organization may be radically different. For example, certain groups of people may not show the usual pattern of

left hemisphere dominance for language skills and right hemisphere dominance for spatial skills. Instead, their pattern could be reversed in part or in total.

2. The pattern of brain organization may be the same but the degree of asymmetry may be less. Some individuals may show a smaller degree of asymmetry because of genetic or experiential factors.

3. The brain organization may be the same, but one hemisphere may habitually be more active or controlling of the person's behavior. In this case, it is not really the brain lateralization that is different, but rather the relative use the person makes of each side.

We will deal with each type of difference in turn.

chapter nine

Is everyone lateralized the same?

If everyone's brains were organized exactly the same, the task of neuropsychology would be simple since there would be no exceptions to the rules. Without exceptions to cloud the issue, the rules of brain organization would be considerably easier to detect. However, such is not the case. Occasionally, there are instances reported of right hemisphere damage causing language disturbance, or of massive left hemisphere damage not followed by aphasia. There are enough of these "exceptions" to warrant looking for factors that can influence the pattern of brain organization. Three have been studied in detail: the hand preference of the individual, early brain damage, and certain early experiences that seem to influence how a person represents cognitive functions in the brain.

HANDEDNESS

What is Left Handedness?

The pattern of brain lateralization described so far is based on the typical right-handed person. However, we know that left-handers comprise from 5 percent to 12 percent of the population, from studies done in North America and Great Britain. There are several factors that influence the census count of left-handers to produce such a wide range.[1]

1. Age—until fairly recently, most or all left-handed children were forced to write with their right hand, leaving only the most determined lefties to represent their group. Thus, there are fewer left-handers in the over 40 years age group compared to under 30 years.

2. Measure of handedness—there are many measures of hand preference, with none universally accepted. Clearly some people have a greater preference than others and the issue is not a dichotomous one. Handedness can be measured on a gradient from one extreme to the other. Because of this vagueness about how to define a left- (or right-) hander, there are reports of from 1 to 30 percent incidence of left-handedness.[2]

3. Cultural pressure to conform—in different parts of the world, and indeed even within countries, the social pressure to conform to the majority right-handedness varies. Rural societies tend to be most conforming, urban less so.[3] The incidence of left-handedness today, considering all the studies, is accepted to be about 10 percent or 11 percent. It is interesting that this overall figure has not varied a great deal over the centuries, despite local fluctuations. For example, Stanley Coren and Claire Porac[4] examined works of art containing active human figures dating back to 3000 B.C. and found a fairly consistent 7–8 percent incidence of left-handedness.

How can we tell whether someone is left- or right-handed? It is not sufficient to just ask, because people often are not aware of the degree to which they use the nonpreferred hand. Sometimes they judge themselves to be ambidextrous when in fact one hand is greatly preferred to the other, and vice-versa. Also, people are not always consistent about which hand they choose to perform a certain task. Thus, a standardized test is needed that is shown to be both reliable (getting the same responses on a second try) and valid (really reflecting what we want to know about). A number of such tests exist,[5] with the most popular items asking about the hand preferred in writing, throwing, using a pair of scissors, using a toothbrush, and drawing.

Handedness and Lateralization

Clinical Studies. With such difficulty even defining left-handedness, it is not surprising that the relationship between handedness and brain lateralization is not clear. However, it is clear there is some relationship because of a number of observations from both the clinic and the laboratory.

First, it has been noted that left-handers do not in general suffer as severe a degree of aphasia from left hemisphere damage as right-handers and their recovery is more rapid and complete. Thus, we presume that language skills are more likely to be bilaterally represented in the brain in left-handers, since language is less likely to be disrupted by damage to one side. In addition, left-handers with left-sided lesions are more likely to show some signs of visual agnosia, spatial disorientation, and dressing apraxia than right-handers, who display these losses only with right-hemisphere lesions, as we saw in Chapter 2.[6]

This is all fairly good circumstantial evidence for a modified pattern of lateralization in some left-handers. More telling are the data from the Wada test (see Chapter 4). Brenda Milner and Theodore Rasmussen have been collecting the results of Wada testing for more than twenty years. As shown in Table 9.1, 96 percent of right-handers show left lateralization for language while the rest show right specialization. In left-handers, the figures are 70 percent and 15 percent, with the remaining 15 percent showing bilateral representa-

TABLE 9.1. Speech lateralization as related to handedness in patients measured via the Wada test (adapted from Rassmussen & Milner, 1977).

HANDEDNESS	NO. OF CASES	SPEECH REPRESENTATION		
		Left	Bilateral	Right
right	140	96%	0%	4%
left	122	70%	15%	15%

tion. The figures for left hemisphere speech in right-handers should be taken as a minimum, as other researchers report almost 99 percent left dominance, also using the Wada test.[7] These figures derive from patients with no signs of left-sided brain damage incurred early in life (as is often the case with patients tested for speech lateralization). Early damage, as we will see shortly, can cause a shift in representation of language to unaffected parts of the brain.

If we accept that these patients did not incur early left-sided brain damage (the signs are not always obvious), we can calculate the incidence of right hemisphere language in left- and right-handers. Considering that about 90 percent of the population is right-handed and 4 percent of these are right dominant for language, about 3.6 percent of the population are right-handers with language primarily represented in the right. About 30 percent of left-handers (who comprise 10 percent of the population) have either bilateral or right-sided language representation, accounting for about 3 percent of the population. Thus, if a person has language represented in the right hemisphere, the chances of his being left- or right-handed are about even.

Experimental Studies. As we discussed in Chapter 4, it is sometimes difficult and dangerous to extrapolate from clinical data to normals. Considering the number of lateralization measures that exist for use with normals, it is not surprising that we have many sources from which to examine the handedness issue. For example, with auditory (dichotic listening), visual (visual half-field) and lateral eye movement tasks, left-handers are less likely to show the usual right side of body (left hemisphere) bias for speech-related tasks.[8] From the results on these measures, however, we cannot specify who has bilateral representation and who is right dominant because the scores on these tests are only approximate correlates of brain organization.[9] As a group, however, left-handers do not produce the same consistent left hemisphere effect on language tasks. Other lateralized skills also seem to be less asymmetric in left-handers: Right-handers show a right hemisphere bias when making judgments about the pitch and loudness of words, while left-handers do not.[10]

Why Should Left-Handers be Different?

Paul Broca originally suggested in 1861 that left-handers all had a reversed pattern of cerebral dominance for language. With such a simple hypothesis—that one hemisphere is dominant for the most important manual and intellectual skills (language)—it is easy to imagine a reason for the effect of hand preference. However, we now know that the situation is not so simple. Several hypotheses exist, ranging from a genetic-anatomical link to an experiential-physiological one.

Genetic-Based Causes.
Some left-handers are left dominant for language, some right, and some bilateral. Is there some way of dividing up left-handers into these three groups that would explain the differences? Three suggestions have been made.

First, the *degree* of left preference may be a factor in determining lateralization and is assumed to have some genetic correlates. There is some experimental evidence with normals that the more strongly left-handed are more likely to be right dominant for language.[11] However, this simple solution was not found in studying the degree of language loss in left- and right-handed aphasics, nor in the hemispheric bias for facial recognition in normals.[12] So this hypothesis requires further work.

A second genetic measure, is *familial sinistrality*—whether or not close relatives are also left-handed. Initial support has come from the incidence of aphasia in familial left-handers, where there is equal likelihood of language loss with left and right brain damage. In non-familial left-handers, there is practically no language loss due to a right-sided lesion, while left-sided damage does produce a loss. Experimental support has been found with both auditory and visual tasks, and sometimes whether there is a history of familial left-handedness is more important a factor than the handedness of the person being tested![13] Familial sinistrality has been implicated often enough to seem important, but not enough for us to be sure of exactly how it ties in with lateralization for language.

A third proposal is that of Jerre Levy and Marylou Reid.[14] Some left-handers write with an "inverted" hand position, holding the pen

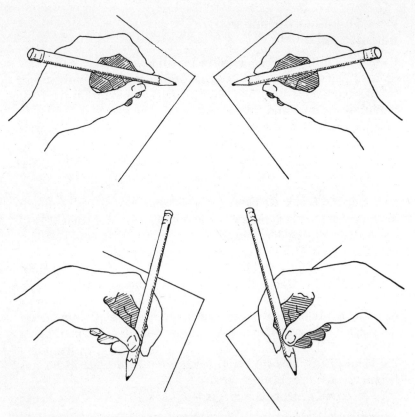

FIGURE 9.1. Levy and Reid (1976) suggest that preferred writing posture reflects brain organization for language, where normal, noninverted position indicates the same hemisphere for speech dominance and hand preference and inverted position indicates opposite hemispheres. Thus, right-handed inverters would have language represented in the right hemisphere, and left inverters in the left hemisphere.

or pencil so that the writing tip points towards the writer (down the page) rather than away (up the page). When asked, left-inverters often say they write like this in order to see what they are writing or (before the advent of ballpoint pens) in order to avoid smearing the ink. However, there are also left-inverters in Israel for whom because of the right-to-left direction of writing Hebrew, neither of these reasons hold! In fact, writing from right to left should cause a dramatic rise in right-handed inverters, but this is not found to be the case (see Table 9.2). Levy and Reid propose that the inverted posture is due to neurological factors, and that this is a sign of "crossed" language dominance where handedness and language skills are not governed by the same hemisphere. They found that in a task of visual lateralization with normals, left-inverters show the same pattern (left hemisphere language dominance) as noninverting right-handers, while left-noninverters show the opposite pattern (i.e. right hemisphere dominance for language). Noninverters, then, would have hand control and language control in the same hemisphere. Right-handed inverters should be rare because at most only 4 percent are right dominant for language. The one inverter Levy and Reid did find showed reversed laterality as expected.

TABLE 9.2. Incidence of noninverters and inverters among left- and right-handers in the U.S. and Israel (data from Shanon, 1978) and in Canada (data from our laboratory). The discrepancy between the figures for Americans and Canadians is probably due to the difference in sample size, male-female ratio (more males are inverters), and different criteria for classification.

LEFT-HANDERS		
	Noninverters	*Inverters*
Americans	36 (60%)	24 (40%)
Israelis	52 (87%)	8 (13%)
Canadians	42 (75%)	14 (25%)
RIGHT-HANDERS		
	Noninverters	*Inverters*
Americans	54 (90%)	6 (10%)
Israelis	58 (97%)	2 (3%)
Canadians	445 (97%)	14 (3%)

Although there is probably something in the writing posture hypothesis, attempts by others to corroborate it have often failed.[15] Also, the number of left-inverters is not sufficient to account for the 70 percent of left-handers who are left dominant for language. Most perplexing is the comparison between Israelis and Americans: There are fewer inverters among the left-handers in Israel, but not a parallel increase among right-handers (see Table 9.2). Probably both biological and environmental factors are at play here.[16]

What Causes Left-Handedness?

We may legitimately ask at this point, what causes left-handedness anyway? There have been a few attempts to account for hand preference using genetic models, where both parents contribute some probability of left-handedness being inherited.[17] The difficulty with these models is twofold: Identical twins who share identical genetic heritage are often (23 percent) discordant for hand preference. Also, almost everyone has a left-handed relative, so the genetic influence model must be very complicated.

Although there are undoubtedly genetic sources, there are also nongenetic sources, both biological pressures and environmental ones. Phil Bryden has built one model allowing for pressures from genetic, nongenetic-biological, and environmental sources. The strength of his model lies in his study of both direction and degree of hand preference in university students and their parents. He found that the preference for left or right hand did not correlate between generations, but the *degree* of asymmetry did. That is, it appears that whether or not one will have a strong or weak hand preference is inherited, but the choice of hand is not. Other biological and environmental pressures generally favoring a right bias may determine this choice. His model is certainly controversial at the moment, but the attractive aspect is that it allows for the many sources.[18]

As briefly mentioned in the last chapter, a physiological factor found recently to be related to handedness is the relative amount of blood flow in each hemisphere. Right-handers tend for some reason to have a greater flow on the right and left-handers on the left.[19] If this difference is present at birth or earlier, it may be a cause of hand preference and may be due to primarily genetic causes or to some developmental happenstance. Admittedly, the difference in blood flow may simple reflect the already present difference in hand preference.

One kind of developmental happenstance that has been suggested as a major source of left-handedness is slight brain damage caused by difficulties at birth. The evidence for this "birth stress" hypothesis comes from a number of sources. First, for a long time people who have worked with children with learning disorders, mentally retarded children, stutterers, and epileptics have noted the higher percentage of left-handers. For example, instead of finding the usual 10–15 percent who are left-handed and ambidextrous, among those special groups the percentage of nonright-handers may be 30–40 percent.[20] Also, it should be noted that these groups contain many more males than females. We know that from conception until death, males are more vulnerable than females for almost all developmental difficulties, both biological and psychological. Perhaps then, the increased left-handedness is also a *product* of such vulnerability. There is no implication here that it is a *source* of the vulnerability.

Does this same principle hold for the normal population? Paul Bakan [21] suggests it does. He has used a relatively crude index of birth stress—on average second and third born children have easier births than first, fourth, and later born—and found that greater stress is related to an increased incidence of left-handedness, suggesting that anoxia at birth (an interruption in the flow of oxygen due to delayed onset of breathing) may raise the level of sinistrality. While we should note that there are difficulties with the data,[22] this principle can in theory account for some of the complications we have discussed so far.

Consider why birth stress might be linked to *left*-handedness. Let us suppose that in 100 births, eight babies experience some degree of unilateral brain damaging anoxia. By chance, four should affect the right hemisphere more and four the left hemisphere more. The ones with left hemisphere damage may have reduced facility with the right hand, thereby developing a left-hand preference. Yet these children were not necessarily "genetic" left-handers, but develop a left preference because of brain pathology. Similarly, there would be right-handers who become more asymmetric because of right-sided damage. Since about 10 percent of the entire population is left-handed, there would be six genetic and the four pathological left-handers. Similarly, there would be eighty-six right-handers without brain damage and four experiencing anoxia. Although the absolute numbers are the same, clearly the anoxic left-handers are going to stand out in their group more than are the anoxic right-handers. This relationship is strengthened by the finding that in monkeys at least, anoxia at birth affects the left hemisphere more than the right. This suggests that there would be more pathological left-handers than pathological right-handers.[23]

Now, if the left-handed group is a mixed one to a greater extent than the right-handed group, it is conceivable that the mixture of brain lateralization found can be due to this. At present, however, we have no way of knowing whether genetic or pathological left-handers are the ones exhibiting the mixed and reversed laterality. The familial sinistrality data do not help because we really cannot tell whether what is inherited is a predisposition to use the left hand or to have difficult birth experiences.

A true test of this hypothesis requires much better birth stress data. Birth order is much too general an indicator. With such data, we might then be able to determine whether pathological left-handedness is due only to severe anoxia, and therefore also associated with psychological and motor problems, or can be caused by very mild anoxia that would not cause behavioral deficits.

The birth stress hypothesis implies that as a group, left-handers have experienced more brain damage and should show intellectual deficits. This is not the case generally. In a large review of all the studies done comparing left- and right-handers in the school system (excluding special classes for slow learners), Curtis Hardyck and his coworkers[24] find no overall effect worth discussing. If there is a deficit at all, it is so small that it would only show up in a very large group average, and still would affect school marks so minimally that no one should be interested in it. Thus, if the birth stress hypothesis is correct, it would have to be either only for very severe cases, so that they would only be in special classes and not in Hardyck's study, or only for cases so mild that no appreciative cognitive deficit would be incurred.

Another suggestion is that specific skills are affected by the bilateral representation of language in many left-handers. As discussed earlier, some claim that since speech is so important, bilateral representation causes other right hemisphere skills to be "crowded out," thereby causing a bias toward verbal skills over spatial skills.[25]

Others claim the opposite, that left-handers as a group show reduced verbal skills and relatively increased visual-spatial skills.[26]

One way to examine the possibility of a difference due to verbal versus spatial skills is to compare the incidence in various professions. For example, there is a higher than normal frequency of left-handers among architecture students with the bias increasing among the advanced students.[27] Similarly, comparing art students at the Massachusetts College of Art and at Boston University School of Fine Arts with undergraduate liberal arts students at Boston University yielded dramatic differences in hand preference,[28] as shown in Table 9.3. However, it is doubtful whether the birth stress hypothesis could account for these results for two reasons. First, there was no difference in birth order between the artists and the nonartists, and second, considering the competition involved in entrance to architecture school and art college the successful students probably do not have a verbal deficit, but rather a visual-spatial talent. It could be that these students are from the 60–70 percent of left-handers with the usual pattern of laterality, the left handedness simply being a reflection of their well-functioning right hemispheres. Among musicians, there are as many or more left-handers as in the general population, even though musical instruments are generally biased against left-handers in their construction.[29]

While we are discussing hand preference, it would be relevant here to consider for a moment the "mixed dominance" hypothesis, which will be discussed in more detail in the next chapter. Some educational psychologists have noted that children with reading difficulties often show an eye preference different from their hand preference. Eye preference refers to the eye preferred when looking through a telescope or microscope, not necessarily the eye with better vision. A difficulty with this theory is that mixed dominance is not unusual, both among children and adults, and therefore can be found in many children without reading difficulties.[30]

TABLE 9.3. Hand preference in artists and nonartists (constructed from Mebert & Michel, 1980).

	LEFT-HANDED	MIXED-HANDED	RIGHT-HANDED
artists	21 (20%)	28 (27%)	54 (53%)
nonartists	7 (7%)	15 (15%)	79 (79%)

THE EFFECTS
OF EARLY BRAIN DAMAGE

One of the traditional maxims of neuropsychology is that if you are going to have brain damage, it is better to have it early. The reason for this is that the chances of recovery are greater in childhood, since it is easier for the functional organization of the brain to be rearranged when still in a less mature state. However, good arguments have been made for the principle that recovery can never be complete because the brain is never the same after damage.[31] Yet, reorganization is more probable if the damage is incurred in infancy or early childhood. For example, Theodore Rasmussen and Brenda Milner recorded by use of the Wada test the side of language representation in patients with definite clinical evidence of early left hemisphere damage (see Table 9.4). Although left-handers are certainly more likely to show speech dominance on the right side, especially after early damage to the left, right-handers as well show an unmistakable shift (compare these figures with those in Table 9.1). Rasmussen and Milner further discuss the type of early damage that promoted the switch in lateralization. In cases where the primary language areas are damaged, there is a high probability of some right hemisphere takeover of speech. When the primary language areas are spared, there is not likely to be a switch, even if the damage is considerable.

Presumably the same principle holds for the representation of other lateralized skills. However, there have been no reports on them for good reasons. Few cognitive functions have primary areas so well-delineated in brain representation as language skills and no other

TABLE 9.4. Speech lateralization determined by the Wada test in patients who sustained early left hemisphere damage (from Rasmussen & Milner, 1977).

HANDEDNESS	NO. OF CASES	SPEECH REPRESENTATION		
		Left	Bilateral	Right
Right	42	81%	7%	12%
Left	92	28%	19%	53%

cognitive skill is so easily tested and as important for continued social existence.

We sometimes take the principle of *complementarity*—if language is represented on one side, visual-spatial skills must be on the other—for granted. Not only has this not been demonstrated in normal individuals (admittedly this is not an easy task), but the early brain damage data suggests it is not correct. Thus someone with right-hemisphere speech due to a fall on his head when he was 2 years old, probably also has right-sided visual-spatial skills. The pattern of lateralization can thus be considerably disturbed by early damage to one side of the brain.

EARLY EXPERIENCES
WITH AND WITHOUT LANGUAGE

We have discussed how brain lateralization effects are due to more than just the physical structure of the stimulus; the strategy and psychological set taken by the individual also affect his asymmetry scores. If these cognitive processes are involved in lateralization, then so too are the experiences that determine which cognitive processes the person uses.

Literacy. Although all people normally acquire a native language, not everyone learns how to read, and literacy may be an important factor in our attitudes and cognitive set concerning language function. However, the exact influence of this factor is unclear. For example, although it is usually left hemisphere damage that produces aphasia, it has been reported that among illiterates right-hemisphere damage is also likely to do so.[32] By this reckoning, a literate language may be more represented in the left hemisphere, or perhaps schooling and the kind of verbal-analytic logic practiced in Western schools promote a left strategy for language. Unfortunately, there are also other reports of no difference in speech lateralization in illiterates.[33] Other varied early language experiences have also been associated with increased right-hemisphere involvement with language. Two involve a lack of speech and a third an abundance.

Lateralization in the Deaf. Congenitally deaf people must communicate using a nonspeech modality such as American Sign Language (ASL). Using the visual half-field technique, deaf subjects have been tested for asymmetric processing ability of ASL signs. To these subjects, the signs are more than just hand configurations—they contain linguistic meaning. Yet there is a lack of left-hemisphere superiority for recognizing ASL signs. Hearing people show a strong advantage for reading English words or letters in the right visual field compared to the left. With ASL hand signs as stimuli, deaf people show no asymmetry while the hearing have a left visual field (right hemisphere) advantage.[34] Signing is a complicated skill involving sequencing skills and grammatical sophistication like a spoken language, in addition to the visual-spatial aspects of the task. It is not surprising, then, that language representation in the deaf might involve right-hemisphere processes as well as left hemisphere activities.

Complicating the situation is the clinical evidence of deaf aphasics who have lost some or all signing abilities. Although only a small number of cases have been documented, it appears this aphasia is due primarily to left-sided damage, just as in hearing individuals. The apparent conflict between the experimental studies and the clinical cases can be resolved by comparing what is measured in the two situations. The experimental studies involve *reading* ASL signs, which have important visual-spatial features. The clinical studies, on the other hand, deal with a loss in active *signing*, a complex manual skill. For this task, considerable manual dexterity and motor movement organization are required, which are skills associated with left-hemisphere functioning,[35] and which the experimental tasks do not require to the same degree. Thus, it would appear that deafness does not alter the organization of language skills in the brain, but the skills involved in the language process may be a reflection of the condition of deafness.

Isolation From Language.   A different kind of language isolation that has also produced right hemisphere speech involves a dramatic case of child abuse.[36] Genie is now a young adult no longer in her dire circumstances, but from late infancy until age thirteen and a half, she was kept isolated, mostly bound to a chair, and deprived of any normal amount of visual, auditory, tactile, and human stimulation. At the time that she was removed by the authorities, she had no language abilities. After a few years of extensive tutoring, she has acquired some language, although her social skills are so poor as to prevent us from knowing whether or not she is capable of learning a standard language. Her pattern of brain lateralization is far from normal for a strong right-hander. She clearly is right dominant for language skills and may be left dominant for spatial skills. Her verbal abilities and thinking style are clearly reminiscent of the capacity of the right hemisphere in normals—very high visual, Gestalt skills, and poor grammatical abilities. It seems that her pattern of lateralization is reversed and she places a great emphasis on what is usually known as a right-hemisphere style.

Bilingualism. From the examples above, it seems that a reduction of normal language experiences results in a reduction of emphasis on the left hemisphere. What about increased language experience as found in bilingualism? Rather than producing an over-reliance on the left hemisphere, the learning of a second language sometimes seems to involve right hemisphere participation! For example, Bella Kotik[37] found that Russians who moved to Estonia and learned Estonian informally show a much reduced left-hemisphere advantage for Estonian compared with Estonians at home who showed an increased left hemisphere advantage on a Russian dichotic listening task. The difference is in the learning. The Estonians learned Russian only in school, the Russians learned Estonian in everyday circumstances.

The situation, unfortunately, is not always so clear since often in different studies no differences are found where they ought to be and vice versa. Also, perplexing cases arise that disturb any neat pattern, such as bilingual patients who exhibit a Broca's aphasia in one language and a Wernicke's in the other.[38] Such cases are, admittedly, the exception to the rule that both languages are affected similarly in aphasia, although one may be considerably stronger than the other. Most perplexing are cases of alternating recovery. Michel Paradis[39] has documented several cases, such as the following:

> The first patient was a 48-year-old educated right handed female who spoke both French (her mother tongue) and Arabic (the language of her work for the past 25 years) fluently before insult. In November 1978 the patient suffered a cerebral concussion in a moped accident in Casablanca (Morocco). Upon regaining consciousness, she was able to speak only some Arabic words. When examined in Paris 10 days later, her French was acceptable but she could not speak Arabic. On the next day her French was very poor but her Arabic quite fluent, and the

following day she was again able to speak French but not Arabic. After discharge from the hospital she was again able to speak French for several weeks but could not find her words in Arabic. Three months later the patient had recovered both languages and returned to Morocco.

The second patient, seen in January 1979, was a 23-year-old intelligent right-handed male who spoke both French (his mother tongue) and English (the language at work for the past 6 years) fluently before the surgical removal of a venous malformation deep in the left parietal lobe. The first language to be recovered for a week was English, and he could not speak a word of French, his mother tongue, to the extent that his father had to act as an interpreter between him and his French-speaking wife. Later, he recovered French, but could no longer speak English, the language of the nurses on the ward. Three weeks later, when the edema affecting the temporo-parietal area had subsided, he was able to speak both English and French again.

That the two languages in a bilingual patient can be differentially affected by brain damage is a strong argument for some separate representation in the brain. However, the exact nature of this separation is still unexplained.

NOTES

1. For reviews of left-handedness see Bryden (1982), Harris (1980), Corballis & Beale (1976), Hardyck & Petrinovitch (1977).
2. Hécaen & Ajuiaguerra (1964).
3. Dawson (1977).
4. Coren & Porac (1977).
5. Annett (1970), Crovitz & Zener (1962), Harris (1958), Oldfield (1971). The last one is currently generally preferred.
6. Hécaen & Sauget (1971); see also portions of Luria (1970b).
7. Rasmussen & Milner (1977); Rossi & Rosadini (1967) give the higher percentage for left dominance, but they do not say whether or not their sample includes cases of possible infantile right-sided damage.
8. Kimura (1967), Zurif & Bryden (1969), Bryden (1970), Kinsbourne (1972).
9. See Satz (1977) for a discussion of this problem of inferring the brain lateralization of an individual from a standard lateralization test.
10. Nachshon (1978).

11. Satz, Fennell & Jones (1969); Shankweiler & Studdert-Kennedy (1975); Lishman & McMeekan (1977).
12. Hécaen & Sauget (1971); Gilbert (1977).
13. Zurif & Bryden (1969); Lake & Bryden (1976); Andrews (1977).
14. Levy & Reid (1976,1978).
15. Moscovitch & Smith (1979); Lawson (1978); Bradshaw & Taylor (1979); McKeever & Van Deventer (1980).
16. Shanon (1978).
17. Annett (1972); Levy & Nagylaki (1972).
18. Bryden (1979a), Bryden (1982); see also Collins' (1977) work with paw preference in mice.
19. Prohovnik, Hakansson & Risberg (1980).
20. See various chapters in Herron (1980); Satz (1972); Bakan (1977).
21. Bakan (1971, 1977).
22. Hicks, Pellegrini & Evans (1978), Schwartz (1977).
23. Brann & Myers (1975).
24. Hardyck, Petrinovich & Goldman (1976).
25. Levy (1969).
26. See Bradshaw (1980) for a review.
27. Peterson & Lansky (1974, 1977).
28. Mebert & Michel (1980).
29. Oldfield (1969).
30. Coren, Porac & Duncan (1981).
31. Isaacson (1975); St. James-Roberts (1979). See also Schneider (1979).
32. Cameron, Currier & Haerer (1971).
33. Damasio, Castro-Caldis, Grosso & Ferro (1976) find the proportion of aphasics among left hemisphere damaged illiterates as among literates; Tzavara, Kaprinis & Gatzoyas (1981) find and even greater right ear advantage in a dichotic listening task among illiterates.
34. Poizner & Lane (1979); Poizner, Battison & Lane (1979); Ross, Pergament & Anisfeld (1979); Scholes & Fischler (1979); McKeever, Hoemann, Florian & Van Deventer (1976).
35. Kimura (1976).
36. Curtiss (1977).
37. Kotik (1979).
38. Albert & Obler (1978).
39. Paradis (1980).

chapter ten

Are some less lateralized than others?

Two right-handed people may differ in their handedness: one may have some agility with his left hand while the other may have next to no dexterity with his nonpreferred hand. The cause of the difference may be biological—with or without genetic factors involved—or may be partly experiential—more practice with the left hand promotes ambidexterity in right-handers. Similarly, some people show a greater degree of functional hemispheric asymmetry than others. We have already discussed how many left-handers seem to have language skills bilaterally represented. There are other factors that have been reputed to affect degree of lateralization. In all cases, the cause of the differences are in dispute—some claim inherent biological sources, others environmental sources.

SEX DIFFERENCES

There seem to be sex differences in almost all important behaviors people engage in. Most likely, many of the differences are just exaggerated stereotypes. However, there are some well-documented differences that are not just necessary results of the obvious biological sex differences in reproductive roles and body shape.[1] Some of these are intellectual, perhaps most cautiously summarized as differences in cognitive style. There is the classic difference, for example, on verbal and spatial skills. Women on average are superior on various verbal and linguistic tasks, and men on some standard tests of spatial ability,[2] although the applicability of those results to the real world is not ensured.[3] Such differences are quite small, are found only as averages in relatively large groups, and are significant only statistically. A number of hypotheses have been developed to explain these sex differences, including genetic models, hormonal models, maturational models, and socialization models. One factor that keeps appearing is brain lateralization: Women show a smaller degree of cerebral asymmetries than men on tests of lateralization, and various researchers have tried to tie together this difference with differences in cognitive skills. Before we discuss these attempts to integrate lateralization and ability, let us review the evidence for sex differences in lateralization.[4]

Although girls show a left-hemisphere dominance for speech as early as boys,[5] there is much clinical evidence that the hemispheres are more equal in language competence in women than in men. For example, Jeanette McGlone found the incidence of aphasia in men after left-hemisphere damage is at least three times that in women.[6] Also, even in the nonaphasic patients, the left-damaged males were significantly lower on verbal IQ than right-damaged, while women show no difference. McGlone also has reported that right-hemisphere damage causes more severe losses in visual-spatial tasks in males compared to females.[7] Somewhat analogous results are also reported for a spatial test with monkeys. Bilateral damage to part of the frontal lobe affects male monkeys at an earlier age than females, suggesting that female monkeys do not demonstrate as great localization of functions as the males.[8]

The experimental evidence with normals is generally not as consistent in indicating sex differences as is the clinical evidence, but when differences appear they point towards greater asymmetries in males. Boys show a greater left-hand advantage than girls on a dichhaptic task for shapes, although the overall accuracy is not different for the two groups, and men show a greater right-hemisphere bias on visual-spatial tasks.[9] Similarly, on verbal tasks (as in reading words, for example),[10] men show a larger asymmetry than women, although the asymmetry is the same for boys and girls from age 5–13 years on a dichotic listening task.[11] When the EEG record on both kinds of tasks is examined, the results indicate greater differences between the hemispheres in men.[12]

The differences in degree of lateralization between men and women are admittedly very small, sometimes only a fraction of the lateralization effects themselves.[13] Yet, they are convincing in that almost always whenever differences are found, they are in the same direction—with women less lateralized. Whether or not this has any significance for differences in cognitive skills will be discussed below. Meanwhile, we can consider various hypotheses accounting for the source of the difference. By examining this relatively small effect, we can expand our understanding of lateralization effects in general.

Neurophysiological Explanations

What can be the source of even small differences between men and women in brain lateralization? One is tempted to consider physiological explanations first, relating the functional differences to some physical differences in the brains of men and women. There is evidence for three sources here: hormonal differences, maturational differences, and anatomical differences.

Hormonal Factors.   The gross anatomical differences between the sexes are induced by differences in hormonal secretion during early development. There has been a long and sometimes acrimonious debate about whether any important behaviors besides those relating to reproduction can be traced to hormonal factors. Generally speaking, environmental factors such as socialization are more easily identified as the responsible influences than are biological factors, although some could argue that this is so only because biological factors are hard to determine.[14] It is especially interesting, then, when hormonal factors *can* be related to behavioral or psychological variables. For example, the degree to which boys show less extreme masculine secondary sex characteristics, such as hip size, shoulder width, and muscle strength, is related positively to scores on tests of spatial ability. The opposite was found in girls, where masculinization was measured by features including narrow hips, wide shoulders, solid muscles and small breasts.[15] In other words, the more androgenous and less sex-stereotyped the physique of the subject, the higher the spatial abilities score. The girls' findings may be related to environmental factors—masculinized girls may more likely be tomboys who play games that may be more oriented towards building spatial skills. But it is hard to see how the boys' results could be accounted for by experience. It would indeed be interesting to have had lateralization scores for these subjects.

The evidence for hormonal factors specifically affecting brain localization of functions is weaker, although a sex difference in a brain function has been detected in monkeys, where female monkeys show less localization of function. The effect can be reversed with an early injection of sex hormones.[16] Hormonal influences in lateralization have not been studied directly in humans, although the link between sex-related hormones and lateralization is striking in some birds. Fernando Nottebohm[17] has been working on the neural substrate for bird song in canaries and zebra finches, of which only the males sing. He has shown that not only is the singing behavior much more tied to brain activity on the left side compared to the right, but also that the cortical regions associated with bird song are much larger in the males. Are sex hormones related to this difference in brain structure and function? Apparently yes, because Nottebohm has found that early implantation of testosterone (a masculinizing hormone) in female birds induces singing behavior and alters the brain structures to be more similar to the males'.[18] This is by no means proof that whatever sex difference in lateralization there is in humans is due to hormone differences, as birds' brains are considerably different from those of humans and this relationship has yet to be demonstrated in humans. Nonetheless, the possibility exists.

Maturation Rate.   Girls tend to mature faster than boys. Also, on average girls score better on verbal tests than on tests of spatial abilities, and on measures of lateralization they seem to show less asymmetry. Are these three factors related? If they are, then the sex differences would more appropriately be called "maturational differences". Deborah Waber[19] found that in both boys and girls, those who mature physically earlier than others also show a considerable bias in favor of verbal over spatial skills. The later maturers have a reversed pattern. Thus, she argues, it may not be that there is any direct link between being male and preferring spatial over verbal skills compared to being female. Rather the relationship is between maturation rate and spatial skill. Since girls tend to mature earlier than boys, these two variables are easily confused. Waber also tested for speech laterality with a dichotic listening test; again she found a relation between maturation rate and degree of lateralization. Among her 16-year-old subjects, the late maturers were significantly more left dominant for speech than the early maturers. Once again, the sex difference in lateralization may be due to maturation rate more than to sex *per se.*

Anatomical Differences. Freud, in reference to sex differences in personality development, once wrote that "anatomy is destiny." We have already seen that the situation is not so clear with respect to brain functions. However, of the anatomical asymmetries that have been found in humans, there are some sex differences to be noted. With respect to the well-founded asymmetry of the planum temporale, which is one of the cortical speech areas, more female brains show a reversed pattern of the right side being larger than males.[20] Other suggestive differences in asymmetries exist, but generally the sample sizes have been too small for us to come to any firm conclusions.[21]

These three neurophysiological approaches are certainly not rivals. They are all compatible with each and are in fact mutually reinforcing. What is it that determines the rate of bodily maturation? Hormones. What influences the rate of growth of brain structures? Hormones. And what influences the pattern of hormonal production? Bodily growth and brain structures. These processes are clearly mutually dependent, a situation reflected in the incredible complexity of the hormonal systems and their interaction with other bodily and psychological factors.[22]

Cognitive Explanations:
Are Sex Differences
More Apparent than Real?

Another approach to the sex differences issue in lateralization emphasizes the point that the differences may be more apparent than real. By this we mean that it often seems that women's brains are more symmetrically organized, while really the sex difference is not in brain lateralization at all. This situation is similar to everyday experiences in other differences among people. Say we compare two people of identical ability, one of whom is more self-confident. Surely that person will *appear* to be brighter at first blush, since some hesitancy in the other's approach to the situation reduces the performance level. Similarly, one might argue that men and women are lateralized in the same way but that women tend to give less asymmetric scores because they approach the lateralization tasks differently. For example, for almost all tasks, one can use various combinations of analytic and holistic strategies, or verbal and visual imagery strategies. Some combination may be more appropriate or efficient than others, depending on the task, but there is no law stating that people must always be efficient. Various environmental pressures may be responsible for sex differences in thinking style that involve more "integration" of strategies in women. Such an integration may be reflected in less asymmetry on lateralization tasks.

Integrating the Visual Environment (Field Dependence). There have been slight but consistent differences found between men and women in cognitive style, especially with respect to *field dependence*, which refers to the tendency to be influenced by the surroundings when making a visual judgment. More discussion of field dependence and lateralization is given in the next chapter. Although the differences are small, as a group men seem to be better than women at isolating a visual stimulus from its surroundings (see Figure 11.1). An alternate way of looking at this is to say that on average, women are more sensitive to the environment. This tendency to visually integrate information could certainly be due to differing patterns of socialization of boys and girls—how often do boys receive comments about how pretty they are or their environment is? A cognitive style integrating the visual environment may generalize to more complete integration of imagistic thinking in other modalities, which would be reflected in more integrated cerebral activities. This highly speculative argument is based on some generalization of the verb "to integrate" from the visual realm to a conceptual one to a neurological one. The validity of this generalization has yet to be demonstrated.

Integrating the Verbal Environment. Little girls are on average more verbal and more socially aware than little boys, a difference variably attributed to socializing influences (parents expect baby girls to be more verbal and social and so talk to them more[23]), to indirect physiological differences (in infancy girls tend to be healthier and so can pay attention to outside stimulation more easily than boys[24]), and even to neurological differences (that the left hemisphere matures faster in girls than in boys[25]). Whatever the source, the result of this situation could be that verbal processes would be less isolated as a specific cognitive domain both intellectually, that is, as a function of the mind, and neurologically, that is, as a function of the brain. Thus verbal skills would be less localized in the female brain and more integrated into all cognitive activities.

Cognitive-Emotional Integration. As we saw in Chapter 2, emotional processes are more tied to right-hemisphere functioning than left. To some extent, emotional and verbal-analytic processes are dissociated in the human brain. However, traditionally the socialized, stereotypical woman in our society is not encouraged to make as great a dissociation, but rather to be the reservoir of feeling in the family. The stereotypical male detaches emotion from action. Clearly these stereotypes are only extremes, but to the extent that they characterize tendencies toward which the sexes diverge (and sometimes strive?), they may be reflected in the differences in lateralization we find between the sexes. If this explanation is indeed true, we should expect a reduction in sex differences in lateralization as our culture becomes less gender-stereotyped, if indeed this is happening. Cultural change would not affect neurophysiological sources, such as hormonal differences.

These environmental approaches do not deny there are sex differences in lateralization *scores*, only that these differences reflect how men and women diverge on thinking styles and strategies. It will be very hard to demonstrate that any of them are correct, although one strategy is to vary style and sex simultaneously and compare them as determiners of degree of asymmetry.[26] The difficulty stems somewhat from the dangerous type of logic used where arguments mix physiology and psychology. The noted neurologist of the last century, Hughlings Jackson, warned against such a mixture; it is all too easy to become sloppy. Unfortunately, keeping neurophysiological and psychological arguments separate is not the point of neuropsychology. It is usually only after the discussion is over that we can look back and see where the unrigorous thinking crept in. On this issue we shall have to wait.

Can Differences in Lateralization Account for Differences in Spatial Skills?

The repeated findings of sex differences in degree of hemispheric asymmetries and in the pattern of spatial and verbal skills tempt one to look for a connection. Despite some attempts to tie all these variables together,[27] we can cite at least three reasons why any relationship would be doubtful.

1. If there were a relationship, then it would be that less lateralization implies lower spatial ability. However, this has not been found to be the case. In a lateralization task of spatial skills, women may identify a more balanced number of items in the left and right compared to men, and still score the same number correct overall.[28] Thus, on the very specific tasks involved in the spatial lateralization tasks, sometimes no difference in ability appears.

2. With auditory tasks (dichotic listening), women tend to show less lateralization only with verbal materials; with the identification of environmental sounds, there tend to be no sex differences.[29] The diminished lateralization for speech in women has been linked to lower spatial skills. Jerre Levy[30] suggests that when speech "takes up" more than the left hemisphere, the spatial abilities that are

usually given full rein in the right are crowded out, either because there is only a finite amount of processing capacity available or because the verbal processes interfere with the spatial activities. However, neither of these has been shown to exist. Presumably, there is some finite processing capacity in a brain (or a half-brain), but until we can better define what is involved in neuropsychological "processing," we will have no idea what this capacity is. If this crowding hypothesis were correct, we would expect left-handers, who tend to be less lateralized for speech as we have seen, also to be deficient in spatial skills. This is patently not the case.[31] Moreover, if "crowding" were a problem, we would expect people who have had only one functioning hemisphere from birth to be highly deficient. Yet they have IQ scores in the normal range, and any specific spatial deficiency is found only when it is the right hemisphere which is missing.[32]

3. There are many tests of spatial skills and it is not clear that they all measure the same abilities.[33] It very well may be that there are differences in particular spatial abilities that are not lateralized, that is, the ability difference is on one type of skill and the lateralization difference is on another. The argument that lateralization and ability must be related is an old one, and will be discussed in more detail with reference to reading skill (see also Chapter 13).

READING DISABILITY
(DYSLEXIA)

As mentioned in the previous chapter, left-handedness and ambidexterity are greater among children with learning disorders, although no causal relation can be inferred. A learning disorder that specifically affects reading skill is called *dyslexia*. The term *dyslexic* is usually reserved for those who have more or less normal intelligence and abilities with the sole exception of reading. Unfortunately, the term is not rigidly applied and so the incidence of dyslexia may be reported as anywhere from 2.5% to 10% of children.[34]

Inadequate Speech Lateralization

Samuel Orton worked with dyslexic children in the early part of this century[35] and recognized the greater incidence of left-handedness among such children. He also noticed a very high incidence of *crossed eye-dominance*, where the person has an eye preference (as described earlier, which eye is preferred when looking through a microscope) different from hand preference. Orton hypothesized that the problem of dyslexia in children stems from a noncomplete dominance for speech of one hemisphere. He also hypothesized that when one reads, the pattern set in each hemisphere is a mirror image of the one in the other. Combining these two ideas, Orton suggested that in children with incomplete dominance, confusion in reading would result because of mirror images of the letters or words intruding from the normally nondominant hemisphere. He also suggested that to detect incomplete dominance, one should look for ambidexterity and crossed eye-dominance, attributes that are very easy to detect.

Orton's theory spurred considerable interest in dyslexia as a specific learning disability distinct from retardation or motivational difficulties, and thus generated a great deal of research on the issue. We are now able to evaluate the aspects of his theory that relate to lateralization, and we now know that the situation is not so simple. First, the hemispheres do not receive mirror image percepts of the environment.[36] Second, crossed eye-dominance turns out to be quite prevalent among normals.[37] Many people with crossed eye-dominance are not dyslexic and many dyslexics do not have crossed-dominance. Similarly, many ambidexterous people are not at all dyslexic. As a screening device, indices of lateral preference fail. Together with this interest in abnormal asymmetry of the brain, Orton placed an emphasis on letter reversals, confusions of *b* with *d* and *p* with *q*. As a symptom of dyslexia, this is inadequate. As has been recently reported, dyslexics do not make relatively more letter reversals than normals although they do make more errors overall. Another characteristic postulated by Orton—that dyslexics are more likely to scan words backwards (right to left)—does receive some support.[38]

This reversal of scanning explains the somewhat conflicting results from other studies that relate to the hypothesis of reduced cerebral dominance for speech in dyslexics. In Orton's day, no tests of brain lateralization existed, except for the retrospective results of unilateral brain damage. Now, however, we can test for lateralization for speech with dyslexics as easily as with normals. The results are not consistent, however, until one takes the scanning issue into account. For example, a popular method involves presenting words to be read in the visual half-field technique. The word is presented either to the left of fixation, to the right, or two different words in both visual fields simultaneously. It is very easy to achieve the appropriate right visual field superiority with this technique.[39] Unfortunately, however, the asymmetry is not due simply to lateralization for verbal material, since the effect of scanning left-to-right should produce the same result. If we accept that dyslexics and poor readers may have as one symptom a difficulty in appropriate scanning habit, the reduced lateralization for speech may be entirely caused by this factor.[40]

On the other hand, tests of speech lateralization using the auditory dichotic listening task are not hampered by the scanning factor. Here, dyslexics do not show less asymmetry.[41] Thus, the principal tenet of Orton's theory, that cerebral dominance for speech is less in dyslexics, has not found favor in modern research.[42]

Inadequate Spatial Lateralization

Another approach emphasizes the specialized functions of the right hemisphere in dyslexics, with an emphasis on sex differences. Sandra Witelson[43] has found that both dyslexic boys and girls are left-hemisphere dominant for speech, as shown by the dichotic listening test. Using dichhaptic and visual half-field tests for lateralization of spatial abilities, she found significantly less asymmetry in dyslexic boys compared to normal boys. Thus, dyslexic boys appear to have less right-hemisphere specialization for spatial tasks. Dyslexic girls, on the other hand, show the same pattern as normal girls—no asymmetry for the spatial dichhaptic task. It seems from these results that lack of right-hemisphere specialization for spatial ability correlates with dyslexia in boys but not in girls, for whom this is the normal state of affairs.

At first, these results seem strange, since it is a verbal skill that is disturbed in dyslexia. However, Witelson reasons this way: Many more boys than girls are dyslexic (up to ten times more).[44] Dyslexics show a verbal deficiency and no spatial deficiency (remember that dyslexia is a term reserved for those who are of normal intelligence).

Although the degree of asymmetry was equivalent on the verbal dichotic listening task, the total number of correct responses was lower in Witelson's dyslexic group, for both boys and girls. On the spatial tasks, the dyslexics showed equivalent total correct, but the boys had reduced asymmetry. The only abnormal aspect of the boys' spatial skills was in their lateralization. For the dyslexic boys, then, the left hemisphere subserves spatial skills to some degree as well as verbal skills. This may lead to the deficiency in reading because, for English at least, spatial strategies are not appropriate, and in these cases the left hemisphere speech mechanisms are heavily imbued with spatial processes. It is interesting to note that children having a very difficult time learning to read English can readily learn to read stories in Chinese ideograms within a few hours—the reading deficiency is restricted to sound-letter correspondence, not whole word correspondence.[45] For girls, mixed cerebral representation of verbal and spatial skills does not pose a problem and we find many fewer girls among dyslexics. There is probably more than one cause of dyslexia,[46] which may account for the existence of some girl dyslexics.

With Witelson's theory, we are left with one piece missing from the puzzle of dyslexia: What is the cause of the abnormal specialization for spatial skills? We discussed earlier in this chapter maturational and hormonal factors that may influence hemispheric specialization. Why, though, should one hemisphere's skills be affected more than the other's? Until this issue is resolved and until her results are confirmed or contradicted in other laboratories, Witelson's theory remains a tentative, if fascinating, integration of several issues in brain lateralization.

NOTES

1. A number of reviews have recently appeared: Maccoby & Jacklin (1974), Wittig & Petersen (1979), Parsons (1980).
2. Maccoby & Jacklin (1974, chapter 3); Harris (1978).
3. For example, Allard (1980) has found that although she obtains the usual sex difference in spatial ability as measured by a standardized test, the sex difference disappears when spatial skill is measured in a test relating to a practiced domain. Male

and female basketball players both do better than nonplayers on her paper-and-pencil test of spatial configurations of basketball players during a game. In other words, a bit of experience may counteract any sex difference in spatial abilities. See Evans (1980) for a short review of the lack of sex differences found when tested in real life situations.

4. Detailed reviews can be found in Bryden (1979b), McGlone (1980), and Harris (1978).

5. Witelson (1976) found a significant right ear effect with 6 to 12 year olds using dichotic listening.

6. McGlone (1977, 1978). Similar unequal sex ratios can be found in Landsdell (1964, 1973), and in an ingenious retrospective analysis, Inglis & Lawson (1981) found that the average degree of verbal versus nonverbal decrement following left versus right hemisphere damage was a function of how many women were in the study: the more women in the sample, the smaller the reported difference.

7. McGlone & Kertesz (1973).

8. Goldman, Crawford, Stokes, Galkin & Rosvold (1974).

9. See Witelson (1976) for the dichhaptic task results; See Kimura (1969), Levy & Reid (1976) for the spatial task; for face recognition and line orientation, see McGlone (1980) for a summary.

10. Levy & Reid (1976).

11. Berlin, Hughes, Lowe-Bell & Berlin (1973).

12. Ray, Morell, & Frediani & Tucker (1976).

13. Not only are the differences small, but they are also usually inferred from reports of men showing a significant asymmetry when women do not. This does not mean that the difference in degree of lateralization between groups is always statistically significant—if men show an average difference of six items in favor of the right ear and women show three, the men's score may be significantly different from zero, while the women's is not significantly greater than zero nor significantly less than six. The correct measure is the statistical interaction between degree of laterality and sex. This is rarely reported, and even more rarely is it significant. Examples of where a difference was found are Lake & Bryden (1976) and Harshman, Remington & Krashen (1975, as cited in Bryden, 1979) for verbal dichotic listening, Kimura (1969) and Levy & Reid (1976) for a visual-

spatial task. A thorough review of where sex differences have been found is presented in Bryden (1982, chapter 15).

14. See Parsons (1980) for a recent debate on these issues.

15. Petersen (1976). See McGee (1979) and Petersen (1979) for reviews.

16. Goldman, Crawford, Stokes, Galkin & Rosvold (1974); Goldman & Brown (1975).

17. Nottebohm & Arnold (1976), Nottebohm (1977, 1979).

18. Nottebohm (1980).

19. Waber (1976, 1977). For a review of these issues see Waber (1979).

20. Wada, Clarke & Hamm (1975).

21. See McGlone (1980) for a review.

22. See Mason (1972) for a review of the complexities of the psycho-endocrine systems.

23. Maccoby & Jacklin (1974), Smith & Lloyd (1978), Frisch (1977).

24. Moss (1967); applying this difference to Sameroff's (1975) trans-actional model, we can see how such a health difference could escalate into a much larger sex difference in parent-child inter-action.

25. The evidence Lansdell (1964) and Nash (1970) present for this argument is only suggestive at best.

26. The fact that lower class children sometimes show less lateral-ization for speech than middle class children (controlling for race), suggests that strategies or motivations can heavily influence lateralization scores (see Geffner & Hochberg, 1971; Geffner & Dorman, 1976; Dorman & Geffner, 1974; and Borowy & Goebel, 1976).

27. For example, Buffrey & Gray (1972) claim that females are *more* lateralized and that this accounts for their verbal superiority and spatial deficit relative to males. Their approach has not found support among other researchers (rather the opposite is now generally accepted), for example McGlone (1980), Marshall (1973). Opposed to Buffrey and Gray's approach is also Levy (1969), who claims lower lateralization implies less ability to keep strategies distinct and so leads to poor spatial skill. We should point out that this assumes a particular solution to the chicken-or-egg question: does poor spatial strategy produce low lateralization or vice-versa? As well, note that lower lateral-ization does not seem to reduce verbal skills in women.

28. For example, see Witelson (1974) for a dichhaptic task.
29. See Bryden (in press) for a discussion.
30. Levy (1969).
31. Even Levy & Reid's (1979) own research showed this: there were no significant group differences in overall scores on the spatial dot localization task.
32. Kohn & Dennis (1974a, b). As Maureen Dennis emphasizes, the performance by hemidecorticates on time-restricted, standard visual-spatial tasks is hampered for physical reasons: the patients are blind in one visual field and paralyzed on one side. Even still, their performance is not anywhere as drastically reduced as one would expect were the crowding hypothesis correct.
33. McGee (1979). Adding to the confusion is the finding that the sex differences, which are only slight when found at all, disappear in some African populations (Jensen, 1975).
34. Corballis & Beale (1976).
35. Orton (1937).
36. Corballis & Beale (1976, Chapter 6 for a discussion of this issue).
37. Coren, Porac & Duncan (1981).
38. Fischer, Liberman & Shankweiler (1978); Pavlidis (1981).
39. McKeever & Huling (1971).
40. Such as in Marcel, Marcel & Rajan (1975), Katz & Smith (1974), Kershner (1977).
41. McKeever & Van Deventer (1975), Witelson (1976); see Witelson (1977b, p. 19) for a review; see Corballis & Beale (1976, pp. 172–174) for a discussion of various conflicting reports using dichotic listening.
42. This has not stopped some therapists from assuming that Orton is correct, devising techniques to "train" the left hemisphere to be dominant, a notion that is certainly not supported by current brain theory.
43. Witelson (1977a, b).
44. On the other hand, Johnson (1973) found that the sex difference in reading skills that favours girls in North America is reversed in Nigeria and not present in England.
45. Rozin, Poritsky & Sotsky (1971).
46. Doehring (1979).

chapter eleven

Are there left and right hemisphere personalities?

It is no news to anyone that different people have different talents, different likes and dislikes. Is it possible to relate these sorts of personality differences to neuropsychological factors, considering that differences in the pattern of brain organization can be related reliably only to factors such as handedness and sex? It could be that there is not an easy way to tie in personality and brain functions. We presume the activity of the brain is related in some way to the person's personality, but there may be no left-right lateral relation.

However, a relatively radical relationship has been proposed involving the concept of *hemisphericity*, which refers to the tendency for one hemisphere to be generally dominant and show greater control over behavior than the other hemisphere. We expect this, of course, in specific circumstances such as during verbal or spatial tasks. Hemisphericity, however, refers to the situation when one hemisphere is dominant no matter what the task. This does not mean the other hemisphere is generally inactive, but rather that the dominant one leads in decision-making. For example, some people may tend to look at the world in a holistic fashion, others more analytically. Each style has its own merits and deficiencies, but it is a rare person who has equal command of both styles and can alternate comfortably. Rather, most people tend to adopt one cognitive style or another.[1] It would be most interesting to be able to match a cognitive style or a personality type to specific hemispheric processing.

"Artist Types" Versus "Lawyer Types"

In our society we have developed what is considered a cultural gap between two styles of thinking. One is characterized by an orderly mentality—epitomized by professionals such as lawyers, accountants, and scientists. The other is characterized (or perhaps caricatured) by an attempt to avoid an emphasis on strict order and logic—as with artists and musicians. There is supposedly a great gulf between them, the one group grasping its cold, analytic, verbal approach to life, the other its emotional, holistic, imagistic attitudes. Within any individual, such extreme personality styles may border on psychopathology. With groups, however, the division makes more sense and it is not surprising that radically different lifestyles and tastes are associated with each.

The two characterizations are highly reminiscent of the cognitive styles associated with the two hemispheres. Following up on this link, a number of researchers have compared various groups on hemisphericity and lateralization, to see whether neurophysiological correlates could be found to differentiate cognitive styles.

First, it should be made clear that we should not expect lawyers and artists to have differently organized brains. On the contrary, we have no evidence to suggest that personality variables determine the pattern of cerebral asymmetries (or vice versa). As far as we know, only the factors of handedness and early brain trauma can affect the pattern of lateralization.

For example, Stephen Arndt and Dale Berger[2] tested eight sculptors and eight lawyers on two laterality measures using the visual half-field technique, one requiring the discrimination of faces, the other of letters. In addition, they gave each subject three tests of spatial-holistic skills and three tests of verbal-analytic skills. As expected, the lawyers tended to do better on verbal-analytic tasks and sculptors better on spatial-holistic tasks. However, both groups showed a right hemisphere superiority for the face discrimination task and a left hemisphere advantage for the letter task. Thus, both groups show the expected pattern of brain laterality. To account for the differences in skill, however, we presume that the lawyers prefer (for whatever reason) to be busy with left hemisphere activities, and are certainly more competent at them compared to the others.

Does this mean that when given a choice, the lawyer types will activate the left hemisphere more than the right hemisphere? Apparently this is the case. James Dabbs[3] has found that while resting, the amount of blood flow to each side of the brain differs for English majors and architecture majors. Using the temperature technique, he found that English majors have a higher level of blood flow in the left hemisphere, and architecture majors in the right hemisphere. Presumably, while resting in a comfortable position, they think about the things they prefer.

Hemisphericity has also been related to as mundane a factor as choice of seating in a classroom. In a study employing the lateral eye movement technique with undergraduate students, Raquel Gur and her associates[4] found that "right movers" and "left movers" tend to seat themselves in classrooms in order to accommodate their preferred direction of gaze, right movers on the left and left movers on the right. Gur also compared choice of seating for those nineteen right-handed students in their sample who sit on different sides of the room for what the investigators classified as verbal and analytic topics (mathematics and natural sciences) versus the more holistic topics (art and social sciences). Eighteen of the nineteen sit more to the left for the verbal-analytic topics, that is, they sit so as to activate the left hemisphere more on these topics (and vice versa for the other topics). Left-handed subjects place themselves almost half and half, indicating no consistent hemisphericity in the group for each topic type. Thus, some students are considered to have right hemisphericity (left movers) and sit in the classroom so as to activate the right hemisphere, and vice versa for the left hemispheric ones. Those who show no overall seating preference choose seats consistent with the hemisphere activation required for that topic.

Field Dependence

Another way of capturing differences in cognitive style involves the concept of *field dependence*: the extent to which an individual's perceptual judgment is affected by the surrounding field of vision. The classic measure of field dependence is the rod-and-frame test. As shown in Figure 11.1, the subject sits in a completely darkened room about twenty feet from a rod and frame apparatus painted with luminous paint. With no other cues besides his own sense of balance to guide him, and with the frame at a distracting angle, the subject must try to adjust the rod to a vertical position by a remote control lever. The task is not easy and the considerable differences in performance that are found between individuals are stable.[5] This test is very similar to the *embedded figures task*, familiar from children's

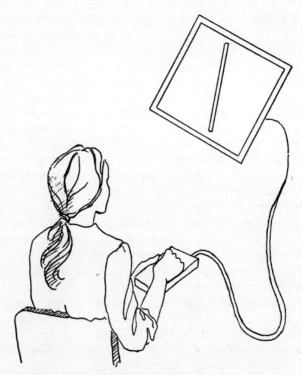

FIGURE 11.1. The rod-and-frame task measures the subject's ability to position a luminescent rod vertically despite the distraction of a nonvertically oriented frame. The room is otherwise entirely dark. The degree of error reflects the subject's *field dependence*.

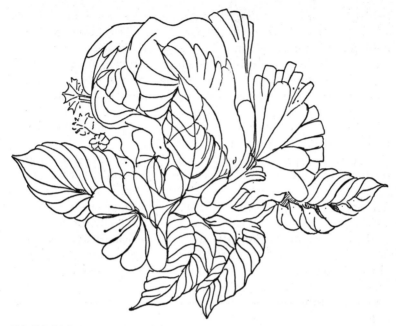

FIGURE 11.2. In an embedded-figures task, the subject has to find a number of some object hidden in a complex scene. In this case, there are 12 birds to find.

playbooks (see Figure 11.2). Both tasks require an ability to ignore misleading and distracting information in order to do well. Performance on this kind of task has been related to brain lateralization in two ways. First, field-dependence could be considered a cognitive style analogous to that of the right hemisphere, while field independence would seem to be a left-hemisphere style. A holistic strategy would certainly produce field dependence errors. Dramatic support comes from a study on patients who were to undergo electro-convulsive therapy (ECT) to one hemisphere for treatment of severe depression.[6] Field dependence scores were obtained before and after the shock treatment, the purpose of which is to disrupt temporarily the normal firing patterns of the brain. In essence, one side of the brain was dysfunctional in the post-therapy test session. In all twelve patients with the left hemisphere temporarily dysfunctional, the errors increased over their pretherapy testing, producing a greater

177

field dependence score. The twelve patients whose right side had been administered the ECT had *improved* scores. They showed *decreased* field dependence. It appears, then, that a more active right hemisphere performs in a field-dependent fashion compared to a more active left hemisphere.[7] Extrapolating to normals, we would conclude that field-independent people would show more left hemisphericity than field-dependent people, who would prefer a right hemisphere mode of functioning, including a predilection for visual spatial tasks over verbal tasks.[8]

Most of the research results have supported, however, another relationship between field dependence and brain lateralization: Field-dependent people tend to show less brain asymmetry than field-independent people. Recall that field independence refers to the degree of differentiation made in the perceptual environment. One could make an analogy to differentiation in the brain's activity. The fact that some people integrate perceptual information more than others (field dependence) may be reflected in the integration of brain functions. In a number of studies, field dependent people have been found to exhibit smaller degrees of brain laterality on the standard tests.[9]

The conflicting results of these two approaches linking field dependence and brain lateralization may be due to a number of factors. For example, the second hypothesis is based on normals, while the first was derived from a psychiatric group, where hemisphericity was manipulated by ECT and field dependence was measured. With the normals, both hemisphericity and cognitive style are naturally occurring, whereas in the psychiatric patients the hemisphericity is imposed. The two groups, then, are not entirely comparable. As with other psychological tests, there may be more than one way to solve the rod-and-frame task. The left hemisphere solution, required by the group with right-sided ECT, may indeed be better but quite unnatural, since analytic (left hemisphere) means are used to solve a normally spatial and holistic task. If this is the correct reason for the dramatic results of the ECT study, we would not expect it to be found also with normals. A second factor complicating the issue is the nature of the concept of field dependence. Is it truly a cognitive style or simply a measure of spatial ability?[10] This is by no means clear and may account for the inconsistent results found.[11]

Other Style Factors:
Hypnotic Susceptibility,
the Television Generation,
and Non-Western Cultures.

A pervasive theme in any review of recent research on brain lateralization has to be the "discovery" of the right hemisphere. As we discussed earlier, the overriding importance of language skills in our society has led to a strong focus on the left hemisphere and its functions, almost to the point where the skills particular to the right side have been left unexplored. The growing awareness among neuropsychologists that the right hemisphere is dominant for many of the more subtle skills has not only clarified for us the organizational structure of the brain, but also reminded us of the importance of these less obvious aspects of thought and personality. The rest of this chapter concerns highly speculative ideas about brain lateralization that emphasize the sometimes hidden contributions of the right side.

Hypnotic Susceptibility. Some people are more easily hypnotized than others. This in itself is not surprising, but it is difficult to say exactly what underlies this difference among people. The search for a straightforward personality trait that is the basis for this ability—for example, degree of acquiescence or neuroticism—has not been successful. There are other skills that do correlate with hypnotic susceptibility: the ability to concentrate, to be absorbed by and emotionally experience a novel, the ability to experience effortlessly some externally directed image or event, as if to globally accept another world.[12]

We do not know what it is that forms the basis for this ability to fantasize, but there are probably some crucial early childhood experiences and some neurological correlates. First, hypnotic susceptibility correlates with the amount of alpha waves produced while resting. This is to some extent a question of relaxation and so may be a reflection primarily of anxiety level.[13] In addition, the concept of hemisphericity has been invoked. All of the skills listed above that are deemed to correlate with hypnotic susceptibility are more characteristic of functions of the right hemisphere than the left. Thus, people who more readily engage in these activities may have relatively more active right hemispheres. Paul Bakan[14] has presented evidence for this hypothesis. Greater hypnotizability is associated with leftward eye movements, an indication of greater right hemisphere activity. Others have found similar results,[15] but there are complicated, inexplicable interactions with sex and handedness, clouding these results.

The ability to become hypnotized probably is related to the state of consciousness while under hypnosis. In Chapter 13, we will discuss the issue of various states of consciousness as related to hemisphericity.

The Television Generation.   Just as we saw that the advent of literacy (Chapter 7) may have altered the functional organization of the brain, the advent of television may also have affected the balance.[16] Although no evidence has been produced to support the arguments, it is interesting to speculate on the possibilities. For the last twenty years, most young children in North America have experienced a massive increase in visual-spatial stimulation early in life, watching events not just in a casual way as one would a street scene, but with the enormous concentration young children are so proficient at giving. Does this stimulation prime the right hemisphere so that it plays a greater part in communication and thought than was the case with the radio generation? We do not know about this possible effect of change within our culture, but the possibility of differences in lateralization among members of different cultures has been explored.

Differences Across Cultures.   To say that profound differences in thought processes and styles of thinking exist across cultural boundaries is only to paraphrase the definition of "cultural boundary." We have already discussed how differences in certain personality traits, abilities, and tendencies have been linked to small yet detectable differences in hemisphericity. It should not be surprising that across wider cultural gaps, we might find differences in lateralization. After all, cultural gaps are no more than differences in cognitive and personality style, differences in focus, and differences in what aspects of life and nature are emphasized. So long as we believe that the brain is indeed the locus of thinking, there must be some relation between differences in brain activity and differences in thinking styles. Although, there is no reason to assume that the neurobiological correlates of cultural differences need be related to hemisphere function, three interesting speculative arguments have been proposed.

The first concerns how the traditional oriental attitude towards life and nature differs from the traditional Western ones. The more holistic attitude of the East sees mankind as an integral part of nature rather than an opponent to nature.[17] The more analytic Western mind places a greater value on verbal forms of logic compared to the more nonverbal holistic ideas. The difference is, of course, highly reminiscent of the differences characterized by the two hemispheres. One could argue that our analytic attitude, divorcing man from nature and thought from things, had its Western beginnings in the fifth century B.C. in Greece with the Atomists, and was developed to a fine art by Descartes in the seventeenth century.[18]

Similarly, anthropologists have been puzzled by the intellectual achievements of some nontechnological societies—not because they expect members of those groups to be stupid, but because some of their achievements are baffling to Westerners and the pattern of achievement and failure can be so very different from ours. For example, the Trukese are a group of islanders in the Pacific Ocean whose sailors can accurately traverse vast distances of open water with seemingly nothing to guide them. The technique they use for navigation is very unlike that of a Western sailor who uses maps to chart his course. The Trukese apparently keep a constantly evolving set of spatial relationships in mind while travelling. Such "relational" thinking contrasts considerably with the analytic, verbal logic that Westerners tend to hold almost synonymous with "intelligence." Indeed, the usual intelligence tests tap primarily analytic logic and not relational thought. Our concepts of intellectual processes ignore thought based on imagistic, noncausal, and contextual logic.[19] These latter types form the basis of the qualitatively different thinking styles of non-Western peoples. The paradox for anthropologists is that while they eagerly accept the notion of qualitative differences in thought processes across cultures, they also assert a basic equality of peoples. This difficulty can be resolved if we consider all people to have within them the two contrasting thinking styles—analytic versus relational, academic versus common sense.

The differences between cultures in thinking styles, some anthropologists claim,[20] is a difference in which hemisphere is dominant generally, the analytic, verbal left, or the imagistic, relational right. The differences that arise, the argument goes, when comparing societies (or individuals) is due to early emphasis on one style or the other.

Perhaps the most audacious attempt to make use of hemisphericity outside the laboratory is that of Julian Jaynes.[21] He has tried to account for why it is that many people hallucinate quite rational voices that give instructions and exhort them to action. Nowadays we attribute such voices to actions of the psychological unconscious[22] and label those who report vivid hallucinations as suffering some mental affliction, such as schizophrenia.[23] The conundrum that Jaynes discusses concerns the prevalence of such hallucinations in the past. Three thousand years ago, he claims, such voices were a part of normal life. People listened attentively for what they considered to be instructions from the gods in times of crisis. Jaynes then says that something happened to Western (i.e. Greek) culture and it became fashionable not to listen to the voices, but instead to self-reflect in order to discover instructions. These voices come, Jaynes hypothesizes, from the right hemisphere, in fact, from the portions of the right hemisphere analogous to the areas on the left that serve language. He asserts that today some altered states of consciousness promote auditory hallucinations in the form of voices, served by the right hemisphere, such as among prophets, poets, in schizophrenia, and during hypnosis. The mechanism is not lost, only suppressed because of a cultural bias against paying attention to such voices.

These last three hypotheses concerning cultural differences in hemisphere functioning are rather extravagant claims. They all make some sense, but are by no means shown to be true. Until empirical work is done to satisfactorily corroborate them, these claims will continue to be considered by experts in the field of brain functions as imaginative science fiction.

Some of the claims can be tested, although little has been done so far to do so. One supportive study of the cross-cultural hypothesis compared speech lateralization in Navajo and Anglo subjects using the dichotic listening paradigm.[24] The Anglos showed the usual right ear-left hemisphere advantage. The Navajos showed the opposite. While these results are suggestive of cultural differences, they are by no means definitive, as the authors realize. However, further studies could be done, for example comparing aphasia rates in various cultures after one-sided brain damage. Similarly, the right hemisphere voices hypothesis could perhaps be examined by EEG analysis in schizophrenics while they are having the auditory hallucinations.

Although fascinating, the free wheeling speculation discussed in this chapter is no substitute for the difficult task of empirical confirmation. Much experimentation is needed before any of these theories can be accepted as beyond fiction. However, neither is experimentation a substitute for imaginative theorizing!

NOTES

1. See Goldstein & Blackman (1978) for a review of literature on a number of cognitive styles.
2. Arndt & Berger (1978). All subjects were right handed men. Similar findings are reported by Dumas & Morgan (1975) and Galin & Ornstein (1974).
3. Dabbs (1980); Dabbs & Choo (1980).
4. Gur, Gur & Marshelek (1975).
5. Witkin & Goodenough (1977).
6. Cohen, Berent & Silverman (1973).
7. Cross cultural support is presented by Dawson (1977) who tested Eskimos and found a relationship among laterality, handedness and field dependence.
8. Berent & Silverman (1973).
9. Oltman, Ehrlichman & Cox (1977); Pizzamiglio (1974); Hoffman & Kagan (1977); Zoccolotti, Passafiume & Pizzamiglio (1979); Zaccolotti & Oltman (1978), Oltman (1979).
10. Wachtel (1972); Widiger, Knudson & Rorer (1980).
11. Negative results are rarely reported in published articles; however I know of at least two failures to find any relation between field dependence and brain laterality: Orr (1980) and Bryden (personal communication).
12. Hilgard (1979), Bowers (1974, especially Chapter 7).
13. Evans (1979).
14. Bakan (1969).

15. Gur & Gur (1974), Morgan, McDonald & McDonald (1971).
16. Debes (1977).
17. Ornstein (1972).
18. For related discussion, see Capra (1975) and Russell (1945).
19. Cohen (1969).
20. Paredes & Hepburn (1976). For reactions from other anthropologists to their proposals, check later issues of *Current Anthropology*.
21. Jaynes (1976).
22. See Galin (1974) for a fascinating discussion on lateralization and unconscious processes. We will discuss this issue further in Chapter 13.
23. For a vivid autobiographical account, see O'Brien (1958).
24. Scott, Hynd, Hunt & Weed (1979). Similarly, Rogers, Ten-Houten, Kaplan & Gardiner (1977) report more right hemisphere activity when Hopi children listen to a story in Hopi than in English. McKeever's (1981) attempt to replicate the Scott et al. findings failed, but of his 20 Navajo subjects, only 13 spoke Navajo and all of these appeared quite assimilated into the Anglo culture.

part five

IMPLICATIONS OF BRAIN LATERALIZATION FOR HUMAN BEHAVIOR

Although the original work on brain lateralization arose from clinical cases, and these results have been extended to normals in relatively narrow experimental laboratory studies, there have been many attempts to relate the differences between the two hemispheres to broader aspects of behavior. In short, do the asymmetries of the brain have any relevance for activities outside the laboratory? It is tempting to extrapolate the research findings to a considerable number of contexts. To be accurate, however, the extrapolations should be as cautious as the original experimental results on which they are based. In order to properly assess where such extrapolations are fair, we will first summarize the various approaches to explaining brain lateralization. The theories discussed represent the main trends and each is based on fairly solid laboratory research. It is clear, however, that none will account for all lateralization effects, and since all these theories are mutually compatible we need not yet reject any.

In Chapter 13, we will see some of the human behaviors that have been related to functional asymmetries between the two hemispheres. In some cases, it may be of interest that the hemispheres contribute differentially in some mental states, such as during hypnosis. In other cases, it may be reasonable to assume that the hemisphere asymmetry plays a causal role, such as with autism, although this has not been proven directly. In still other cases, the issue of brain asymmetries has entered the sociopolitical arena, where society and school systems are exhorted to change in order to more harmoniously match the potentials of the two hemispheres.

In Chapter 14, we will discuss another very major theme in psychological theories: why people do (sometimes strange) things without conscious motivation. *Dynamic* theories of psychology claim there is a part of us of which we are aware (our conscious selves) and that there are parts of us of which we are unaware (our unconscious selves). When we try to delve into this supposed unconscious self, we fail and most of us deny that such an entity could exist. Dynamic theorists respond, "Of course! The point of the hidden self being unconscious is that it is *un*conscious. You can't get at it directly in the same way as you get at other information about yourself." We should keep in mind, as do clinical psychologists, psychiatrists, and social workers, that sometimes people do things that are out of keeping with the conscious self we are familiar with. Could there be lurking beneath the surface another set of needs, desires, and abilities that are usually only manifested in very subtle ways? This dissociation has been mapped onto brain lateralization as a mechanism. We will see that with this extrapolation, there is much to be done before it will be founded in fact.

chapter twelve

Theories of brain lateralization: what underlies hemisphere asymmetries?

There is no doubt that there are functional asymmetries in the brain. Can we point to a simple general distinction that summarizes the asymmetry? Is there a single concept or small set of concepts that captures the essence of what it is that makes one hemisphere different from the other?

There have been many such attempts, the first ones simple and based on observable behavior. For example, from the clinical literature, cerebral dominance for language overrides all other factors. There is a verbal and a nonverbal hemisphere. However, even the earliest neuropsychologists knew that this rather global dichotomy would have to be replaced with some finer level of analysis. We have already discussed in Chapters 5 and 6 what about language might predispose the left hemisphere to be dominant for that function. In this section, I want to explore further some of the different approaches to explaining brain lateralization in terms of more general theories. These theories are neither comprehensive nor mutually exclusive. However, they give some idea of the range of possible answers we might get when we ask why the brain reacts in an asymmetric way to some tasks.

THE PROCESSING OF SPEECH

One of the most robust laterality effects is the dichotic listening task with consonant-vowel syllables. Let us examine some properties of speech that may hold the clue to the left hemispheric superiority on this task.

Some Characteristics of Speech Sounds

Speech sounds—sounds produced by the human vocal apparatus and used in language—have a number of acoustic characteristics that differentiate them from other sounds produced in our environment. For example, human speech includes several bands of sound at various frequencies as is seen in Figure 12.1 The concentration of sound around a particular frequency is called a *formant*, and there may be two, three, or more distinctive formants for a particular

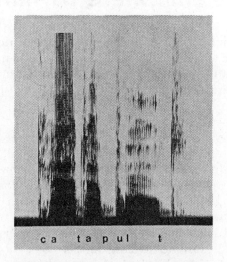

FIGURE 12.1. The sound spectogram shows the strength of sound at each frequency interval (the vertical axis) over time (the horizontal axis). Notice the formant transitions and changes in each syllable of the word catapult.

sound. The band of sound at each formant has a certain width encompassing a range of frequencies. Human speech produces a fairly wide bandwidth with concentrations at the formants. Pure tones, for example, have very narrow bandwidths; musical instruments a variety of acoustic properties (see Figure 12.2). In Figure 12.2, we see sound structures for the thud of a book falling on a table, and a human whistling and humming the same note. Besides speech having characteristic formant structure and bandwidth, there are characteristics of formant changes during speaking. For example, in Figure 12.1 we see the changes involved in going from one phoneme to the next in the word *catapult*. These *transitions*, as they are called, are critical for the encoding of speech. As we saw in Chapter 5, certain sounds are coded acoustically in a complex fashion. Notice how the *d* sound has different formant structures depending on the vowel that follows it (see Figure 12.3). Some sounds like *b* are not constant and their formant transitions are dependent on the vowel context (notice that you can't say a *b* without putting some vowel after it, however short it may be). These encoded sounds are the consonants *b, p, d, t, g,* and *k*. These six consonants differ from each other in terms of two factors: *place of articulation* (where the air is released, be it from between the lips, from between the tip of the tongue and the roof of the mouth, or from between the back of the tongue and the roof of the mouth) and *voice onset time* (how soon the vocal chords start moving after the release of air). See Figure 12.4 for the voice onset time distinction. The sounds *b, d* and *g* involve a voice onset time of about 10 to 20 milliseconds, while their counterparts *p, t,* and *k* usually take at least 40 milliseconds.

This has been a quick review of a number of characteristics of speech. Some of them are not arbitrary since languages other than English involve similar acoustic properties, and newborn babies seem to recognize some of the sounds. For example, the voice onset time boundary at 25 milliseconds produces two classes of consonants recognized by adults around the world. Place of articulation, however, varies considerably from language to language. All languages have the additional properties of wide bandwidth, formant transitions, and rapid changes in the signal. Could some of these factors be responsible for the left hemisphere representation for language?

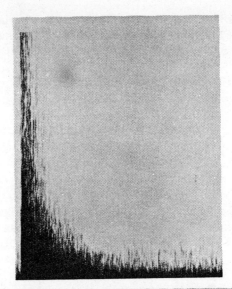

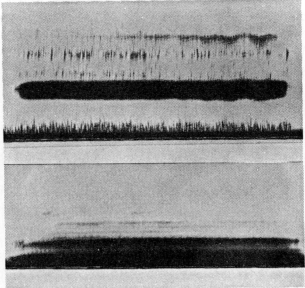

FIGURE 12.2. Here are spectograms illustrating the varying sound structures of a thud (a book falling on a table), a person whistling and humming the same note.

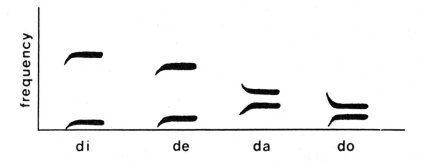

FIGURE 12.3. The same consonant does not produce the same formant structure in different vowel contexts, yet we perceive the consonant as constant. Such consonants are referred to as *encoded*. In this diagram, the formant structure is simplified to accentuate the effect.

In Chapter 5 we saw some of the evidence given in favor of this approach. Let us review this evidence and consider what kind of theory of lateralization we would be left with.

Voice Onset Time.   Voice onset time has been well studied for two reasons. First, it is a factor easily controlled in experiments. With the advent of computer-generated and computer-edited speech, it is possible to produce whatever voice onset time is needed. Second, there is a universal quality to the distinction, in that it is recognized around the world, by prelinguistic infants, and even by another species—chinchillas.[1] Naturally, it is a good candidate for left-hemisphere representation, but the evidence is against this. Dennis Molfese found with average evoked response analysis that not only do both hemispheres seem to distinguish short from long voice onset time, but that another component of the averaged evoked response differentiates the two classes of sounds in the *right* hemisphere only. He surmised that perhaps this distinction is not a linguistic one but rather a general acoustic one. If this were the case, then the same result should be found without having to use speech materials. Using computer generated tones, he found that *tone onset time* is a distinction the right hemisphere makes independent of the left, although this does not mean the left does not also appreciate onset time.[2] Thus,

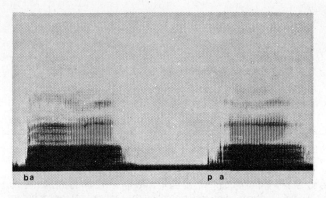

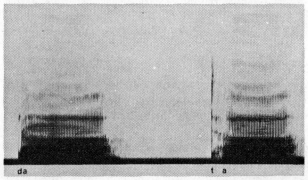

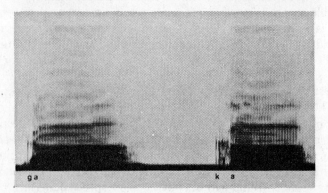

FIGURE 12.4. Voiced stop consonants (b, d, and g) have an earlier onset of vocal chord movement than the unvoiced ones (p, t, and k).

although onset time is important in human speech it is not a factor predisposing language to be left-lateralized.

Place of Articulation. Although the sounds *b* and *g* each have a variety of formant transition structures, we nevertheless perceive them to be constant over contexts. We recognize a *b* as *b* wherever it occurs, and herein lies a mystery for the field of speech perception. One way of seeing whether the ability to perceive the invariance is lateralized is to present these consonants in several contexts. Molfese did just this while recording evoked responses and found that despite the varied contexts—before the vowels *ee* (as in beet), *a* (as in bat) and *o* (as in bog)—the consonants *b* and *g* produced distinctions, but only in the left hemisphere.[3] Place of articulation, then, seems to be a well-represented linguistic mechanism in the left hemisphere. That this factor and not voice onset time should be left-lateralized fits well with a study with aphasics. They were found to have significantly more difficulty differentiating place of articulation than voice onset time compared to normals.[4]

Formant Transitions. The process involved in distinguishing formant transitions also seems to be left-hemisphere based. There are right ear (left hemisphere) advantages to reporting stimuli that differ only in formant transition in the dichotic listening paradigm.[5] Similarly, averaged evoked responses differentiate formant transition differences in the left hemisphere only.[6]

Bandwidth. In a dichotic listening study, only wide bandwidth speech-type sounds produced a right ear advantage. Stimuli (also computer generated) with a bandwidth of only 1 cycle per sec (1 hz) but the same format structure did not produce an ear asymmetry. Thus, it appears that the bandwidth may be a crucial factor in left hemisphere representation.[7] Unfortunately, the difficulty with this conclusion is that the narrow band stimuli did not sound like speech while the wide bandwidth stimuli did. Keeping in mind that whether or not the subject treats the stimuli as speech can affect the ear advantage (see Chapter 5), we can see that the effect is not firmly settled.

Implications For a Theory of Lateralization. If it is some acoustic property of the speech code that predisposes language left-lateralized, we would expect these effects to be universal and to be present fairly early in development, perhaps even at birth. But what about all the other lateralization effects we have discussed so far? They could be seen, perhaps, as byproducts of the original asymmetry. For example, since language depends on speech, the linguistic functions of syntax and semantics would become similarly lateralized. If this is the case, then we would expect these nonspeech functions to become associated with the left hemisphere but not irrevocably tied to that side. Thus, the identification of words not based on speech sounds (as with nonalphabetic codes) should show less of a left hemisphere bias. This is the case with Japanese Kanji, ideograms not based on the sounds of the words. Whether or not this is so with sign language for the deaf is not yet clear.[8]

Other cognitive processes that are asymmetrically represented would, by this scheme, be left-sided if they were very involved in language processing and right-sided if not. Examples of these are given below in the next sections. Some language-related processes may be so basic to thinking, however, that both hemispheres would represent this information. For example, the relationship between the agent and the object of an action (often the subject and object of the verb in a sentence) is represented similarly in the two hemispheres.[9] This is clearly an important grammatical concept, but also goes well beyond language.

FINE MOTOR AND PERCEPTUAL PLANNING

In Chapter 6, the possibility was raised that the left hemisphere's superiority in dealing with speech rests on its advantage in making fine timing discriminations. In a variety of studies using the dichotic listening paradigm, a right ear advantage arises when fine temporal distinctions are required. These may be for judgments of time between click presentations or identification of phonemes with longer than usual formant transitions.[10] Fine temporal distinctions are crucial, of course, for speech as well as for other activities.

More generally, though, let us consider the notion that it is the left hemisphere that plans movements, and that left-sided damage disrupts such planning generally to a greater extent than does right-sided damage. We explored this idea somewhat in our discussion of apraxia in Chapter 2 and of the evolution of lateralization in the previous chapter. To review briefly, Doreen Kimura has found that left hemisphere-damaged patients not only are deficient on linguistic tasks, but also on coordinating a sequence of simple manual movements.[11]

If we extrapolate to the speech domain this notion of planning being left-hemisphere based, once again we arrive at a basis for language dominance. Going further, though, we can appreciate the vast amount of organization required in language behavior, beyond that needed to simply get the phonemes together correctly. These coordinations at various levels can be disrupted by aphasias due to left-sided damage. For example, speech planning is obviously disrupted in Broca's aphasia, due to damage in the left frontal region. The coordination of word output, getting the rhythm of the sentence correct, is also basic to human language and can be disrupted in transcortical motor aphasia due to anterior left frontal damage. As mentioned in Chapter 2, the disruption of meaning relationships is seen in semantic aphasia, due to left-sided injury of the area joining the parietal, occipital, and temporal lobes. In this syndrome, the patient appears to understand the words said, but cannot coordinate the relationships intended. For example, the patient cannot decide which should go on top given the instruction "Put the red block on the blue block."[12]

Although this approach to brain lateralization will account for language dominance, it is hard to see how all other effects fall within this framework. After all, fine visual judgments do not favor the right visual field (left hemisphere) unless they are for some specific element in the figure. Surely the visual tasks that favor the right hemisphere, such as recognition of faces, line slants or clockfaces, require fine discriminations. It may be that there is a difference in magnitude in the fineness of the discriminations the hemispheres are most adept at, the right being better when the discrimination is more global. This idea is at the core of the approach in the next section. To return to organization of actions for the moment, though, the split-brain studies militate against such an explanation. The isolated right hemisphere is much more adept at constructing a specific design from blocks than is the left. Thus, the right hemisphere representation of nonlinguistic functions may have to have another explanation if we accept the approach of this section.

COGNITIVE STYLE

Any attempt to characterize the difference between the hemispheres produces a dichotomy: the left is like this, the right is like that. We can work at a fairly basic level, examining behavior closely to see what cognitive skills are required and to find neuropsychological bases for them. At some point, however, it is tempting to raise our distinctions to a more grandiose level and call them cognitive styles. Thus, rather than say the left hemisphere is more adept at dealing with formant transitions in speech, we say the left brain is verbal and the right is nonverbal and visual-spatial. Certainly, we are now talking at a behavioral level with which we can empathize. The danger is that once we have a label for a cognitive style, we are very tempted to extend our thoughts on the nature of brain lateralization to include some logical extrapolations from the label.

It is certainly useful to be able to make a generalization that goes beyond the explicit data that gave rise to it. Indeed that is why we have theories. But it is important to keep in mind that statements on cognitive style differences between the hemispheres are just extrapolations. The purpose here is to examine the source of these ideas. We should avoid here the simple verbal/visual-spatial dichotomy because it refers to the content of the difference rather than to a mechanism underlying the content. Besides, we have already discussed the difference in some detail.

Analytic Versus Holistic.   Some material must be broken into elements in order to make sense. For example, a sentence consists of words which have relationships; a new word in English must be parsed into units in order to be sounded out. On the other hand, sometimes a global approach is appropriate. The individual lines in a Chinese ideogram convey no meaning by themselves, and the emotional tone of a sentence is not a series of patterns that have meaning in themselves. These two ways of examining or appreciating the world are complementary and have been mapped onto the left and right hemispheres. For example, Tom Bever and his colleagues asked subjects to lift a finger off a telegraph key when they heard a target item in a list of syllables. The target was either the entire syllable or only the first phoneme of the syllable. They found a right ear advantage only for the phoneme detection. They conclude that "the left hemisphere is dominant only for tasks that require analysis of the internal structure of the stimulus."[13] A similar finding is reported in the visual domain. In our laboratory, we found a right visual field (left hemisphere) advantage to reading and playing musical chords on a keyboard. Musical notation is obviously a spatial code, yet the task is analytic in that the individual notes must be decoded to give the response.[14]

This characterization of the left hemisphere being analytic in nature while the right is holistic has been pushed a long way in accounting for lateralization results. Face recognition, as we saw in the Ross and Turkewitz study in Chapter 6, produces a right hemisphere advantage when global features are attended to, and a left hemisphere advantage when the subject's strategy is analytic. Similarly, when subjects use an analytic strategy for remembering a melody, the left hemisphere is involved, while a more global strategy prompts a right hemisphere advantage.[15] Production of speech requires some analytic activity, such as the piecing together of appropriate word and sound units. Comprehension of language allows various strategies to some extent, and it is not odd that the right hemisphere can comprehend some words and commands.[16]

This analytic-holistic distinction, when coupled with the verbal/visual-spatial contrast, gives us the stereotype so often touted in the popular press: The left hemisphere is verbal and logical (and therefore unimaginative and stodgy) while the right is imaginative and irrational (and therefore creative, fun, and usually repressed). It should be clear by now that this characterization is very far from the data. The traits of logic, creativity, and fun really stem from the land of extrapolation I warned about earlier.

Other Style Dichotomies. There are other style differences attributed to the two hemispheres that are somewhat similar conceptually to the analytic-holistic one. For example, it has been suggested that the verbal proclivity of the left side is due to the fact that it processes information serially, which suits speech quite well, while the right side tends to process input in parallel.[17] This maps onto the analytic-holistic distinction very well.

In a similar vein, the labels *focal* and *diffuse* have also been applied to the processing and organization of the left and right hemispheres. In this scheme, the diffuse organization of the right side predisposes it favorably to visual-spatial processing and a holistic attitude.[18]

Implications of Cognitive Style for a Theory of Lateralization. With a cognitive style approach, a thought process is asymmetrically represented in the brain to the extent that it relies on one style or the other. Thus, if the same task can be done using a different strategy, employing a different style, that task can be seen to be variably lateralized. The issue is not, then, whether or not the processing of speech or visual material is lateralized, but whether or not the cognitive operations the subject applies to the input favor one hemisphere over the other. Considering the processes that are needed to properly deal with speech as a language signal, we should expect a left-hemisphere dominance for speech. Given the cognitive style approach alone, I find it hard to see how the neonatal lateralization data can be accounted for. But of course, this approach is not incompatible with the other theories, and they may each have a grain of truth to them.[19]

NOTES

1. Lisker & Abramson (1964), Eimas, Siqueland, Juscyk & Vigorito (1971), Kuhl & Miller (1975).
2. Molfese (1978b, 1980b).
3. Molfese (1980a).
4. Miceli, Caltagirone, Gainotti & Payer-Rigo (1978).
5. Darwin (1974), Cutting (1974).
6. See Molfese (1978a), although the formant transition effect in this study may instead be due to the place of articulation distinction, which is entirely confounded with it.

7. Cutting (1974).
8. Ross (1983).
9. Segalowitz & Hansson (1980).
10. See Efron (1963), Schwartz & Tallal (1980), Robinson & Solomon (1974), and Mills & Rollman (1979.)
11. Kimura (1977).
12. Luria (1969). See Chapter 2 for a fuller discussion on these syndromes.
13. Bever, Hurtig & Handel (1976).
14. Segalowitz, Bebout & Lederman (1979).
15. Bever & Chiarello (1974), Gordon (1975).
16. See Chapters 2 and 5, and Gazzaniga (1970).
17. Cohen (1972). I should point out that although by necessity speech production is a serial behavior, there is clearly much overall structure to speaking that defies a simply linear description.
18. Semmes (1968).
19. See Segalowitz & Gruber (1977b and c) for further discussion.

chapter thirteen

Is brain lateralization related to specific mental conditions?

So far, we have discussed how the two sides of the brain are associated with different capacities and preferences. Not surprisingly, people have related the duality of the brain to particular conditions of mind, some abnormal and some normal. In this chapter, we will discuss some of these applications. Some of them are reasonable, but others are founded more on hopeful dichotomizing than on scientific evidence.

ABNORMALITIES OF FUNCTIONING

Reading Disability

One of the first general applications of brain lateralization in this century was to the problem of reading disability in children. As mentioned earlier, Samuel Orton was interested in children with learning disabilities and he noticed that many children with reading difficulties read words in reversed order. For example, *was* might be read as *saw*. They also sometimes wrote backwards, so that the result would be a mirror image of the intended word. Often these children showed an unstable hand preference. He concluded that there is a link among these symptoms mediated through an incomplete cerebral dominance for language. There are major difficulties with the theory, as described in Chapter 10.[1] Despite this, the idea that there is less cerebral dominance in children with reading disabilities has remained popular, and in many studies dyslexics and normals have been compared on lateralization. Some of these were discussed earlier. The upshot of these studies is that no consistent difference in cerebral asymmetry can be found, yet there clearly is some verbal deficit in dyslexics.[2] Thus there is a functionally deficient verbal component, probably in the left hemisphere, but no convincing evidence that the problem is due to or related to abnormal cerebral representation of language.

Stuttering. More positive, although tentative, results have linked stuttering to hemisphere asymmetries. The idea here, similar to Orton's concerning dyslexia, is that there are competing language centers in each hemisphere, or that at least there is some right-hemisphere mechanism that interferes with smooth left-hemisphere execution of speech. For example, in one report four stutterers who had bilateral speech according to the Wada test improved after surgical removal of one of the speech centers. Similarly, in a brain blood-flow study involving two stutterers, both showed greater blood flow over Broca's area on the right during speaking while simultaneously having greater left flow in Wernicke's area. When the two patients took a drug to alleviate the stuttering, the blood flow was greater for both areas on the left side.[3] Thus, at least in these cases, it appears that competition between the hemispheres is related to stuttering.

Autism. Autistic children are socially aloof, use deviant language, and often engage in repetitive behavior. For many years this syndrome was seen as having social parameters. The children were not considered retarded or brain damaged, but to be suffering from some psychodynamic problem. Now, however, there is considerable evidence that autism is at least partially due to brain damage or dysfunction,[4] and it has been suggested that the dysfunction is characteristically in the left hemisphere. There is behavioral

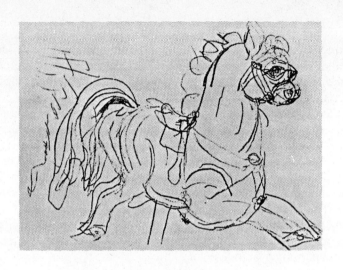

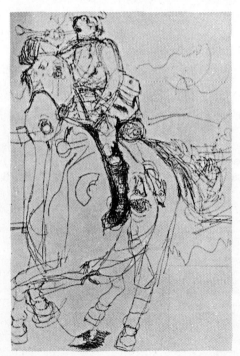

FIGURE 13.1. Nadia is an autistic girl with amazing drawing ability. The horse was drawn at 3½ years of age and the bugler at 5½ years. From Selfe (1977). Reprinted by permission.

evidence to support this notion. For example, some autistic children show an extraordinary affinity for art or music. In one dramatic case, a girl named Nadia showed classic autistic symptoms, yet made incredible drawings (see Figure 13.1). As therapy (and perhaps age) alleviated her autistic symptoms, especially her uncommunicativeness, Nadia's drawing skill diminished.[5] Her drawing style was one of quick movements, almost as if without premeditation, yet they produced considerable accuracy. Similar stories abound of autistic children with a single highly-developed talent. Although the talents range from music to calendar calculation, a characteristic common to them is the speed and lack of reflection in their execution.[6] In some ways, this is reminiscent of the holistic processing style attributed to the right hemisphere.

Other research supports this conclusion. For example, there is an abnormally high percentage of nonright-handers among autistic children. Instead of the usual 10–15 percent who are left-handed or ambidextrous, among autistic children the figures are 50–65 percent. Moreover, autistic children prefer to listen to both stories and music with the left ear, while normal children tend to use the left ear for music and the right for stories,[7] findings also suggestive of a left-hemisphere dysfunction. More direct than these data are those comparing autistic children with retarded children matched for I.Q., and with a group of bilaterally brain damaged children. On a test battery designed to detect brain damage, the autistic children showed evidence of left-sided damage compared to the other two groups, but relatively normal right hemispheres.[8] Since, however, autistic children do not resemble left brain-damaged children (they are neither aphasic nor hemiplegic), the deficit may be a functional one, where the left hemisphere does not function as it should. We will see in the next chapter that this notion has been used for other disorders as well.

ALTERED AND ORDINARY STATES IN NORMALS

Altered States: Hypnosis and Dreaming

The idea that one hemisphere can be more activated during certain tasks and that the two hemispheres serve different functions has been invoked to account for a number of specific states in normals. Some states other than normal consciousness, such as hypnotic trance and dreaming, are so different from ordinary consciousness that physiological concomitants are assumed to be striking, if only we can find them. Some researchers have tried to link these altered states to changes in hemispheric activation.

For example, in a hypnosis study, subjects did a dichotic listening task before, during, and after hypnotic induction. As shown in Figure 13.2, the degree of asymmetry dropped considerably during the hypnotic trance. Because the measure used adjusts for total response accuracy, the difference cannot be due simply to poorer performance during the trance.[9] The authors suggest that this indicates a change in cerebral laterality during hypnotic states. More likely, the data suggest that there is either a change in relative hemisphere activation (the right side becoming more active) or a shift of attentional bias to the right hemisphere during the relaxed state.

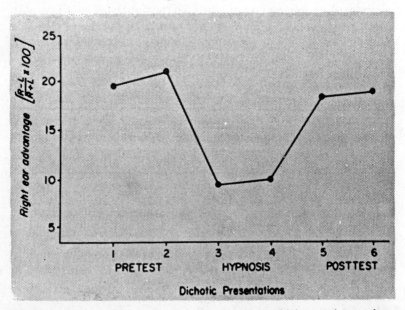

FIGURE 13.2. The degree of left hemisphere dominance (right ear advantage), as measured on a dichotic listening task with consonant-vowel-consonant syllables, reduced considerably during hypnotic trance. From Frumkin, Ripley & Cox (1978) Reprinted by permission.

Considering the confounding of attentional bias and cerebral dominance effects in the dichotic listening paradigm used (see Chapter 15), it is difficult to decide which interpretation is correct.

The duality of the brain has also been implicated in dreaming, although the argument for the link is tenuous. There were early reports of patients who, after suffering localized brain damage, no longer had dreams. The idea of dreaming depending on the integrity of some particular brain region seemed reasonable.[10] However, the reports were relatively anecdotal: Patients would say that they did not recall any dreams. We know, however, that despite five or six dream periods each night, people normally recall only one or two or often none at all. In order to obtain fuller dream reports, subjects must be awakened during or immediately after a dream episode. Such episodes can be detected by monitoring ongoing EEG and rapid eye movement (REM) activity. Using such a procedure to test the specific hypothesis that dreaming is a right hemisphere activity, some researchers have found that split-brain patients do report dreaming and the content of the dreams. Thus, the left hemisphere does have access to dream material in these patients.[11] In cases where there is a loss, then, the problem may be one of recall rather than actual experience.

Rather than considering dreaming *per se* to be a right hemisphere function, it may be more fruitful to look at the content of dreams. Dreams are laced with visual images and emotional ideas. For this reason alone, we should expect a greater right hemisphere participation in most dreaming. In fact, considering the free reign these thought processes are given in dreams and how restricted and controlled they are during waking states, it is not at all odd that several researchers have suggested that Freud's notion of the primary process (the psychological representation of primitive, instinctual needs) should be linked to the right hemisphere.[12] Consider the content of dreams of split-brain patients. Klaus Hoppe, a psychoanalyst, did a detailed analysis of the dreams of twelve split-brain patients and found that they did indeed recall them, so the isolated left side (presumably the language dominant one) does have access to them. They were not of the usual sort, however. The

content of the dreams reflected reality, affect, and drives. Even in the more elaborate dream, there was a remarkable lack of distortion of

> latent dream thoughts. The findings show that the left hemisphere alone is able to produce dreams . . . [P]atients after commissurotomy reveal a paucity of dreams, fantasies, and symbols. Their dreams lack the characteristics of dream work; their fantasies are unimaginative, utilitarian, and tied to reality; their symbolization is concretistic, discursive, and rigid.[13]

Thus, it appears there may be a lack of communication between the left hemisphere and the source of imagery and fantasy. Although daydreaming is not disrupted, Hoppe reports an abnormal lack of symbolized fantasy. Is it fair, then, to conclude that the unreal fantasies and images one experiences at night depend on right hemisphere functioning? It is tempting to say so, but we must remember that the data come from epileptics who have undergone major brain surgery. Until it is shown that these two factors cannot be responsible for the effect, we must hold judgment on the issue. Ideally, data will be forthcoming that will link the content of dreams in normals with patterns of asymmetric EEG activity.

Normal States

Education and the Right Hemisphere. Hemispheric asymmetries have also been called upon to provide a neurophysiological foundation for a wide variety of normal behaviors. Workers in this field, in fact, often delight in collecting examples of the strange extrapolations to which hemisphere asymmetries have been applied in the popular media. There are claims for a considerable range of endeavors for which the forgotten right hemisphere is supposedly dominant, from wine tasting to a contemplative lifestyle. I once heard an earnest young woman explain that marathon swimming allows her repressed right hemisphere to, you know, do its thing. It would be a rather interesting dichotic listening or EEG asymmetry testing procedure that would provide scientific support for hemispheric activation while swimming.

More seriously, we can examine a number of claims made about brain lateralization and everyday behavior. For example, is there a relationship between creativity or insight and hemisphere asymmetry? It has been suggested that the right hemisphere is responsible for intuitive thinking, and that to be most creative one should let the left hemisphere "listen" to the right and act on its results. The complaint is that our public schools traditionally rely too heavily on a left hemisphere-based curriculum emphasizing only verbal skills, while our society devalues the right hemisphere intellectual strengths generally.[14] Is this really something to be concerned about? Undoubtedly, the traditional three R's rely on verbal skills and analytic thinking, and over the last two decades there has been much debate over how broad the school curriculum should be.

It very well may be that a diverse curriculum with some emphasis on nonverbal skills leads to a better-educated child. However, the arguments in favor of a well-rounded education should not invoke brain lateralization. Such an argument draws implicitly on the notion that the brain and mind have similar developmental properties (not just relatable structures). One such implicit notion is that the brain needs exercise for healthy and complete development. However, there is no neuropsychological data to support the notion that one can exercise the brain and train it as one would a muscle. While we speak of "exercising the mind," mental gymnastics of a specific sort do not necessarily make for healthier brain function. It is true that in grossly deprived environments, rats and other animals have been shown to have abnormal brain development (presumably inferior). But in these studies, the comparison is between nearly no stimulation at all versus a very active environment, not a choice between relatively reasonable curricula. Moreover, these studies mainly concern visual stimulation, which may produce changes in the visual cortex, but the content of the stimulation has not been shown to be relevant.[15] Rather, we should judge the value of a varied curriculum by the results it produces.

If we accept the appeal to neuropsychology, the logical extension is preposterous: Every brain has a cerebellum, therefore physical coordination should be included in the curriculum: likewise, eating, sleeping, aggressive and sexual behavior have brain correlates. To allow every brain area to exercise its functions simply means to encourage all possible behaviors. Surely one need not use a neuropsychological argument to support the idea of a balance between physical and mental exercise. The ancient Greeks raised this ideal without reference to brain function. Neither does the fact that there is localization of function in the brain support or deny a particular school curriculum. We should keep in mind that there are many ways to learn, and although restricting a curriculum to only one learning style is unnecessarily limiting, restricting it to only two may also be unwise.

Professional Choice and Hemispheric Balance. Is the choice of profession one makes related to the asymmetrical functioning of the brain? Recall the study discussed in Chapter 11 about hemisphericity and lateralization of sculptors and lawyers. Although the groups clearly differed in the strength of relative skills (verbal versus spatial), the pattern of brain representation was the same. Could it be that the pattern of relative skills is due to some brain determinant? At the moment, we really cannot answer this question. Any one of three logical possibilities may be true and there is not much basis on which to support any of them over the others.

1. It may be that one hemisphere's strength (not yet defined except in circular terms[16]) is focused on because of inherent biological factors. A "strong" hemisphere may be dominant generally, encouraging the person to use one cognitive style over another.

2. It may be that one hemisphere becomes more efficient or dominant through practice, where the decision to practice a skill is made for nonbiological reasons, such as reinforcement or availability.

3. A third possible relationship between hemispheric representation and skill level is that the choice may be only one of mind, not brain, and that no permanent changes accrue from extra use of one hemisphere's skills. This situation would be very much like that in a computer. Repetitively using a set of routines located in one part of the memory bank will not cause changes in the hardware of the computer. "Exercising" the addition algorithm does not make that routine more efficient or healthier.

Why do Notions of Laterality Get Overextended?

Overextension of lateralization constructs is a serious problem in the field. We may legitimately wonder why the problem seems to be greater here than with other fields of scientific study. The answer probably stems from the attractiveness of the dichotomy model. For

TABLE 13.1.

ANDERSON	Expression	Perception
BOGEN	Propositional	Appositional
BOGEN & GAZZANIGA	Verbal	Visuospatial
BRUNER	Rational	Metaphoric
FREUD	Secondary process	Primary process
GOLDSTEIN	Abstract	Concrete
GUILFORD	Convergent	Divergent
HEAD	Symbolic or systematic	Preceptual or non-verbal
HOBBES	Directed	Free or unordered
JACKSON	Propositionizing	Visual imagery
W. JAMES	Differential	Existential
A. JENSEN	Transformational	Associative
LEVI-STRAUSS	Positive	Mythic
NEISSER	Sequential	Multiple
OPPENHEIMER	Historical	Timeless
PAVLOV	Second signalling	First signalling
POLANYI	Explicit	Tacit
PRIBRAM	Digital	Analogic
PRICE	Analytic or reductionist	Synthetic or concrete
RADHAKRISHNAN	Rational	Integral
SECHENOV (LURIA)	Successive	Simultaneous
SEMMES, WEINSTEIN, GHENT, & TEUBER	Discrete	Diffuse
WEISENBERG & McBRIDE	Linguistic	Visual or kinesthetic
J. Z. YOUNG	Abstract	Map-like
ZANGWILL	Symbolic	Visuospatial

Dichotomous terms have often been used to describe different modes of intelligence. This list of authors and their terms come from a larger set compiled by Bogen (1969; 1977).

centuries human endeavours and feelings have been described on linear continua. Table 13.1 provides an easily-extendible list. The great advances of the past two decades in biology and medicine tempt us with biological models for almost everything, which is not odd since there must be a biological basis for every human activity even if that basis is trivial.[17] The notion, therefore, of the two hemispheres representing the two ends of some favorite continuum is often too attractive to ignore. Whether or not there is rigorous evidence for the particular dimension in question sometimes becomes a side issue. We cannot overemphasize, though, the importance of this issue. The difference is one between fanciful hypothesis and supportable theory.

To return for a moment to the issues raised earlier in this chapter, it may turn out that there is a relative shift in hemisphere activation level during relaxation. This would account for the hypnosis effect. It would also account for the relative difficulty of getting right hemisphere effects during vigilance tasks, such as in visual half-field presentation. But in any case, even when such effects are reported, they are found to account for a surprisingly small amount of the variation in scores. Most of the differences between the various psychological states are, as far as we know, due to other factors besides differential hemisphere activation.

Even more important, before we even argue about adapting school curricula or lifestyles to be more compatible with this model of the brain, the effects should at least be demonstrated reliably. Imagination, intuition, and creativity have not been linked to brain activity in any direct experimental work, and, to repeat, even if they were, it is not a logical necessity that they should be pertinent to the school system because of that link.

NOTES

1. See Corballis & Beale (1976) and Rourke (1978) for summaries and critiques of Orton's (1937) approach. Naylor (1980) discusses some of the difficulties in the experiments comparing lateralization in poor and good readers.
2. McKeever & VanDeventer (1975), Gordon (1980).
3. Jones (1966); Wood, Stomp, McKeehan, Sheldon & Proctor (1980).

4. Rimland (1964), Damasio & Maurer (1978).
5. Selfe (1977).
6. Rimland (1978).
7. See Colby & Parkison (1977) for the handedness data, Blackstock (1978) for the ear preference study.
8. Dawson (1981), Dawson, Warrenburg & Fuller (1982).
9. Frumkin, Ripley & Cox (1978).
10. Humphrey & Zangwill (1951). See Galin (1974) for a review
11. Greenwood, Wilson & Gazzaniga (1977).
12. Galin (1974), Bakan (1978).
13. Hoppe (1977, pp. 232–234).
14. For example, see Dirkes (1978) and Bogen (1977), but see also Katz (1979) and Hardyck & Haapanen (1979).
15. Rosenzweig (1979), Greenough (1975).
16. That is, suppose skill X is superior to skill Y; X is associated with say, left hemisphere functioning; why is the person stronger in X? Because the left hemisphere is more efficient than the right. How do we know the left is stronger than the right? Because X is superior to Y.
17. This biological reductionism is easily seen in the misapplications of genetics to behavior (cf. Rose & Rose, 1973; Wahlsten, 1979).

chapter fourteen

Hemisphere asymmetries in psychodynamic processes

I do not love thee, Doctor Fell,
The reason why I cannot tell;
But this alone I know full well,
I do not love thee, Doctor Fell.
THOMAS BROWN (1663-1704)

As we discussed briefly in Chapter 6, there is now the serious possibility of there being a physiological counterpart to different aspects of the psyche, a separation of intellectual and emotional components of the mind. In a now-classic paper published in 1974, David Galin outlined a framework for a theory that links the right hemisphere to unconscious processes and the left hemisphere to conscious thought.[1] The idea is that the verbal behavior of the left hemisphere is clearly conscious and so is in the center of the conscious aspect of self. The right side, however, is not as much in contact with the language mechanism of the other side, and so can initiate thought patterns that are not fully recognized by the left, conscious half. The term "conscious" is used here to denote that which the person can report, material to which the language mechanism has access. This does not

mean the right hemisphere is incapable of thought or even consciousness (used in the broad sense). It is capable of desires, ideas, and
plans as we saw in Chapter 3. Recall the split-brain subject whose
right hemisphere had its own goals and opinions. Rather, Galin
suggests those thoughts that are unconscious are primarily right
hemisphere based. These thoughts are conscious when they make
contact with left hemisphere mechanisms (as very many do in
normals). In the split-brain patient, the reason for the lack of contact
is obvious. When the right hemisphere initiates behavior, the left side
tries valiantly (often in vain) to make sense of the situation. It is
accurate to say that in this case a part of the split-brain patient's mind
is acting independently of the part that dominates the social interaction. In the normal person, such behavior that could not be
explained adequately by the language hemisphere would be
considered to have origins in the unconscious.

Clinical evidence for this notion can be found in cases of
hysterical paralysis. Most often it is the left side that is incapacitated,
implying that the right hemisphere is responsible for the symptom.[2]
In this situation, it may be that some psychological processes that are
active mainly in the right hemisphere are reacting strongly to some
frustrating condition. What could these frustrated psychological
processes be? Therapists would point to emotional needs that are not
satisfied. When these needs are listened to and assuaged, sometimes
through psychotherapy, the person has learned to attend to them. We
can then say the person is "in touch with himself." This "being in
touch" may have neurophysiological correlates in lateral communication between the hemispheres.

How Many Selves are There?

When we talk of a verbal-rational self and an emotional self, we could
also list other components of mind: a visual-spatial intellect, an
aesthetic self, a self sensitive to biological needs, and so on. To the
extent that these systems are functionally independent, we each have
within us a group of selves. Of course, this is the traditional
approach of psychodynamic theorists. Freud explicitly listed three,
the id, ego, and superego; Jung preferred a whole array of archetypes.
For these psychologists, mental stability requires becoming familiar
with the various aspects of our psyches so that each can be afforded its
appropriate expression.

What could be the brain correlates of such a system of selves? Gazzaniga and LeDoux, as we saw before, talk about the system in sociological terms, as a sociology of mind. In their model, each self vies for control, and behavior becomes the complex integration. Suggesting separate compartments in the brain for these selves runs into the problem of mixed metaphors, of ascribing a neurological substrate for a psychological construct. But there may be something about the function of each hemisphere that differentially involves it in the kind of behaviors that these constructs were created to describe.

How do They All Work at Once? When a person experiences something, the entire brain reacts to the stimulation. This can be seen, for example, with evoked responses in the EEG that spread across the entire cerebrum. The response to a visual stimulus can be found all over the surface of the brain, despite the probability that the EEG waveform characteristic to the stimulus is generated in one brain area (for example, the visual cortex).[3] So if there are functionally separate selves, each presumably reacts to all stimulation in its own way. They can be thought of as separate members of a team. At what level do the members act together as a team? This is the critical question for a lateralization model of psychodynamics. Gazzaniga and LeDoux claim that it is at the level of overt behavior that the systems communicate.[4] Thus, the emotional self may initiate some affective reaction, such as crying or feeling happy, and leave the other components of mind to figure out what happened. Often the responsible event is obvious and we detect no separation of selves. Other times, the reaction seems uncalled for at first blush, one might say, and the inability to trace the origin may cause consternation. In any case, the source must be ferretted out, and the discovery may be illuminating. This independence and simultaneity of affective and intellectual reactions is well documented in behavioral psychology.[5] It is the neurophysiological link that is now intriguing.

Evidence for a Right Hemisphere Basis to Emotional Experience

We have discussed some of the experiments with normals indicating a greater right hemispheric participation in emotions.[6] In addition, there are studies of right brain-damaged patients that found they have difficulty comprehending the mood of the speaker while dealing well with the content. For example, they would fail to recognize that a commonplace sentence, such as, "The boy went to the store" said in a gruff, loud voice conveys an angry mood. Similarly, the expression of emotions by means of intonation cues may be disrupted by right-sided damage.[7] Also, right hemisphere damage is more likely to induce "la belle indifference," an indifference to and even denial of illness, despite objectively obvious symptoms such as hemiplegia. The patient may, for example, explain away a paralysis of the left arm by claiming that he does not feel like moving it, that he is tired, and so on.

Another linkage of the right side of the brain to emotional states is more indirect. It has now been reported quite often that depressed patients who have no brain damage, when given a battery of neuro-psychological tests, come out with a profile similar to that of patients with right-sided damage. The performance of the patients returns to normal as the depression lifts.[8] To the extent that a similar profile may indicate a similar dysfunction, it is possible that at least some affective disorder can be linked to right hemisphere dysfunction. A dramatic, if odd, case of this was described by Lewis C. Bruce in 1895. A Welsh sailor with a manic-depressive psychosis was bilingual in English and Welsh, and right-handed when manic, and unilingual in Welsh and left-handed when depressed. There is no question of lateralized damage here. Rather, this is a case for shifting cerebral activation.

Positive Versus Negative Emotions. For several decades, neuropsychologists have noticed in cases of unilateral brain damage different changes in mood associated with each side. For example, although only a minority of patients show such strong reactions, when the patient does experience a "catastrophic" reaction he is much more likely to have sustained a left-sided lesion. A catastrophic reaction includes intense anxiety, crying, swearing, a refusal to cooperate, and a renouncement of the testing situation, without mention of the obvious complaint—a right-sided paralysis. In contrast, an indifference reaction includes being indifferent to failure, joking fatuously, explicitly denying the illness including the hemiplegia or minimizing the symptoms, and attributing them to weariness or drug injections. These are overwhelmingly associated with right-sided lesion.[9]

Similar reports have been given about a patient's reactions to the Wada test. During the brief period when the sodium amytal begins to lose its effect, the patient with a left-side injection expresses a depressed attitude, generalized worry, and a sense of guilt. Right-side injection has been reported to produce a euphoric reaction, smiling, laughing, and a sense of well-being.[10]

These data imply that when the right hemisphere is incapacitated in some way, the left side produces an unrealistically happy disposition. Similarly the right side is depressive when the left's activity is disrupted, implying some mutual inhibition when both are healthy. To call the left side happy-prone and the right sad-prone would oversimplify and miss the point of the investigation. What is it that accounts for the differences? Could it be something about the holistic approach of the right hemisphere that predisposes it to depression? Is the analytic approach of the left hemisphere an inducement to be happy-go-lucky? Or rather, is it the partly incapacitated hemisphere that is producing the reaction? Until we can answer these questions, the situation will remain unclear.

Affective and Schizophrenic Disorders as Lateralized Abnormalities

In the last few years, a rather bold hypothesis has emerged concerning psychopathology and brain lateralization. Affective psychosis, meaning clinical depression in the main, has been linked to right-hemisphere dysfunction, while left-sided abnormalities have been linked to schizophrenia. Schizophrenia is a term used to describe several sorts of nonemotional thought disorders. Delusions and flattening of affect are among the major symptoms. Schizophrenics often show an obvious disturbance of language, so much so that fluent aphasics are occasionally misdiagnosed as schizophrenic.

The evidence for the divergent lateralization of the syndromes comes mainly from three sources. The first involves lateral EEG differences in each group. For example, there are reports of excessive left-hemisphere activity (high-frequency EEG) in schizophrenic patients. Similarly, there is considerable variation in the averaged evoked response over the left hemisphere in such patients.[11] Complementing this, Don Tucker and his colleagues induced depressed and euphoric moods in normal subjects (through hypnotic-like suggestion) while recording EEG activity. They found a reduction of alpha activity (indicating greater activation) over the right frontal lobe during depression compared to the left side. This difference was significantly greater than the asymmetry found in the euphoria condition, where there was basically no change. Thus, depressed mood is accompanied by an increase in right frontal activation.[12]

The second source of evidence concerns a deficit in schizophrenics in the efficiency of transmission across the corpus callosum. In other words, it is suggested that schizophrenics have difficulty communicating between the hemispheres and that therefore the left side's bizarre activity is due to incomplete information. Of course, the poor communication could equally be a result of left hemisphere overactivation. In a series of studies, schizophrenics showed relatively poor transmission of information, for example, when matching two objects, each felt by only one hand, or when verbally reporting something identified by the right hemisphere via the left ear.[13]

The third tack taken on this issue involves looking at indirect measures of hemisphere functioning. Pierre Flor-Henry argues that a left-right difference in hemispheric involvement in schizophrenia versus affective disorders can be shown by relative differences in verbal and performance IQ. For example, he reports a relative drop in verbal IQ scores with schizophrenics, while affectively disordered patients show no such drop.[14]

Difficulties With the Model. Despite the impressive arguments in favor of the lateralized deficit model, the data are not all that clear. For example, the asymmetric activation data bring up some dilemmas to dispel. If depression is related to an *overactive* right frontal lobe, why should nonbrain-damaged depressed patients mimic right frontal *damage* on neuropsychological tests? Is the increased activation of an inhibitory nature, a disrupting influence? If so, the similarity to brain damaged patients' profiles could be understandable. Until this issue is cleared up, it will remain very difficult to interpret the findings.

There is a severe problem in this field with replication. Many researchers produce apparently contradictory results.[15] I use the word "apparently" because the testing situation is very complicated. For example, the definition of schizophrenia includes a list of symptoms, certain combinations of which lead to the classification. This means that some patients may be called schizophrenic with a set of symptoms somewhat different from the set for others. Across studies, then, the subject populations may vary considerably. Even more serious, though, is the problem of drug maintenance. In the battery of drugs given to psychiatric patients, there may be many that are responsible for the effects discussed. For example, it is not hard to imagine that some drugs would interfere with similarity judgments of two objects felt by different hands. Thus, when a problem of inter-hemispheric transfer does occur in schizophrenics, is it due to the drugs that are administered to them but not to the control group? On this same issue, it should be noted that split-brain patients with next to no interhemispheric communication do not seem schizophrenic at all.

The indirect evidence from verbal and performance I.Q. tests is the most difficult to interpret. Schizophrenia is a condition known to include a language disturbance. But also, it is a condition that drastically impairs interpersonal communication. Timed movements, on the other hand, may not be so affected in schizophrenia as in depression. It is not odd then to find an interaction between syndrome and verbal versus performance I.Q. The difference need not be related to hemisphere dysfunction.

The model clearly raises many unanswered questions, and much more research is needed before we can accept the linkage of psychopathological disorders with lateral brain dysfunction. A correlation has yet to be firmly produced. If one does exist, though, we must be careful to examine whether or not a left hemisphere dysfunction simply reflects the symptoms of the syndrome or really gives us an understanding of the nature of the deficit.

Why the Right Hemisphere for Emotion?

The experimental evidence is clear: The right hemisphere is more proficient at identifying emotional stimuli, such as facial expression and tone of voice. As discussed above, the clinical evidence supports this conclusion. Right brain-damaged patients are more impaired in identification and appreciation of emotional tone. When it comes to feeling positive versus negative emotions, there may be some differentiation between the hemispheres, but this has yet to be systematically demonstrated in normals. So why the right side for emotions? We can ask this question in much the same way as we asked it for language and the left hemisphere. Indeed, we may even get a similar answer: because a conspiracy of factors supports this association.

The right hemisphere has been characterized as being more holistically inclined than the left, as more of an integrator, and more comfortable with visual images. Each of these factors is important in emotional perception and perhaps even in emotional behavior. Holistic perception encourages an appreciation of the relationships within the stimulus. For example, a smile does not indicate happiness if the forehead suggests worry, by being wrinkled. An integrative process keeps attention on many factors that each play a part in building the emotional experience. In the experimental tasks that demonstrate a right hemisphere bias for identification of emotions, such as dichotic listening for crying, shrieking, and so on, or such as visual recognition of emotional faces, imagery plays a large part. Thus, there may be a conspiracy of factors contributing to the right hemisphere basis for emotion. Note how purely linguistic or analytic tasks make relatively little use of these processes.

Another accounting for the link involves a developmental explanation. Just as was argued earlier that a faster-developing right hemisphere would predispose it to dominate in the infant's treatment of its early visual environment, that hemisphere would be more likely to deal with the other most important aspect of the infant's life—its affective ties. One could argue that the child's first interactions with the world are affective, and the first weeks and months are spent developing an emotional bond to those caring for it.[16] A faster-developing right side might then become dominant for this function, and since this is the dominant function for much of the child's behavior (that is until language gains control), the right hemisphere may play a leading role in behavior for the first few years. After that, it may regulate and feed content to the left hemisphere; a proper, balanced interaction between the two hemispheres bodes well for a balanced mental life.[17]

NOTES

1. Galin (1974).
2. Ley (1980b), Galin, Diamond & Branff (1977).
3. John (1971).
4. Gazzaniga & LeDoux (1978).
5. Zajonc (1980).
6. See Chapter 6. Also see Galin (1974) and Tucker (1981) for summaries of research on this topic.
7. See Heilman, Scholes & Watson (1975), Tucker, Watson & Heilman (1976) and Foldi, Cicone & Gardner (1983) for disturbed perception of emotions; see Tucker, Watson & Heilman (1976) and Ross & Mesulam (1979) for disturbed production.
8. For example, Bruder & Yozawitz (1979). Related to this result is the finding that when electroconvulsive shock therapy (ECT) is given to relieve the symptoms of depression, ECT when given to the right side is more effective than when given to the left (Galin, 1974).
9. Gainotti (1969, 1972).
10. Terzian (1964) and Rossi & Rasadini (1967) report the positive results. On the other hand, Milner (1967) did not find any evidence. Whether or not this difference in results is due to the first author's dealing with Italian patients while Milner had Canadian patients is unknown.
11. Flor-Henry (1976); see Roemer, Shagass, Straumanis & Amadeo (1978) for the evoked response work. Much of this research has been collected in Gruzelier & Flor-Henry (1979).
12. Tucker, Stenslie, Roth & Shearer (1981). Different asymmetric activation is also implied for depression versus schizophrenia in lateral eye movement studies (Gur, 1978, 1979).
13. Dimond (1979), Dimond, Scammell, Pryce, Huws & Gray (1980). A much-quoted finding lending support to this notion is that the corpus callosum is significantly larger in schizophrenics, presumably making the transfer of information more difficult

(Rosenthal & Bigelow, 1972).
14. Flor-Henry (1976).
15. See Gruzelier (1979), who summarizes many of the contradictions in the field.
16. Erikson (1963) calls this first period one of building a basic trust about the world, a very emotional concept. Giannitrapani (1967) argues for a right dominance because of this.
17. See Ley & Bryden (1981) for a further discussion of the role of emotion in consciousness.

part six

SOME ISSUES
FOR THE FUTURE

In this introduction to brain lateralization, we have so far reviewed the field with an emphasis on positive findings. Having attained a general perspective, we should, before we close, present some of the difficulties in doing lateralization research. These difficulties are not simply technical, although there clearly are enough of those. Rather, there are conceptual, sometimes philosophical issues that determine how our research is designed and therefore what kind of results we are limited to finding. As a research enterprise, the field of brain lateralization has graduated beyond the initial stages where almost any positive result was interesting. Now, a result must be conceptually illuminating as well, and to be so, some of these conceptual issues must be addressed.

chapter fifteen

When is an asymmetry not an asymmetry?

In the early days of experimental neuropsychology, it was exciting enough just to find a systematic asymmetry in behavior. Such a result was taken to indicate that the two sides of the brain function differently. However, the novelty of that finding wore off after a while. People started to ask for some details: Is it the case that only differences in hemisphere functioning can account for the asymmetry? At what level of processing does the asymmetry appear? What parameters control the asymmetry? In this chapter, we will explore some of the issues that put a check on runaway enthusiasm for lateralization. An asymmetric score on some lateralization test *can* be a result of processes other than the hemisphere differences we have discussed so far.

Artifacts of Lateralization Procedures

So far we have accepted asymmetry results as an indication of functional differences between the hemispheres, limiting examples and references to studies that control as best possible the artifacts we are about to discuss. Naturally, researchers in the field have discovered a number of pitfalls to be aware of, some obvious, some not so obvious. For example, if the stimuli going into the two ears in a dichotic listening task are not of identical loudness, the louder one is perceived better. Similarly, in the visual half-field paradigm, the stimuli must be matched in size, brightness and lighting. There are, however, more subtle artifacts of the experimental procedures.

Artifacts in the Dichotic Listening Procedure.

Recall that in the dichotic listening procedure, the subject hears competing messages in each ear and is expected to report or react to them. Immediately though, we see there are quite a number of choices to be made about the procedure. How many items should be presented to each ear on a single trial? Should the subject simply report whatever is heard best? Should the subject attend to one ear on half the trials, and to the other on the rest? If the subject reports at will, should we score which ear he chooses to report from first as well as the correctness of the item? These questions may sound picky, but they do reflect problems in the interpretation of dichotic listening results.

Remember, the idea in this procedure is to obtain some hemispheric advantage for speech reflected in a superior performance with one ear compared to the other. Could a person have a bias to favor the right ear for reasons other than left-dominance for speech? There are several reasons for answering yes to this question. For example, right-handed people may attend to their right side generally. The right bias may encompass more than dexterity. In the original study validating the dichotic listening procedure, Doreen Kimura had both left- and right-handers in both of her left and right language dominant groups. The left-dominant group tended to show a right ear advantage, the other group a left ear advantage. Yet within these groups, left-handers favored the left ear and right-handers the right ear, so that there is a handedness effect as well as a speech dominance effect.[1] Ear advantage can be due to more than speech dominance.

Similarly, a person's ear asymmetry may be affected by the reporting instructions. If allowed to choose which ear to report first, the subject may be biased towards one, which automatically puts the other ear at a disadvantage. The memory requirement for the second stimulus reported is considerably harder than for the first. Asking subjects to attend to a particular ear produces a more stable effect by reducing this variation due to the subjects' ear biases.[2]

Let us assume we have a procedure in which the asymmetry truly reflects differences in processing between the hemispheres, and that our stimuli are linguistic. It is not straightforward to conclude that the ear asymmetry is an accurate reflection of speech dominance. As mentioned in earlier chapters, there are ways that other factors can influence the result. Consider, for example, the study where syllables were presented dichotically and the vowels in them were to be identified. In one condition, the syllables were embedded in a larger series of speech sounds. A right ear advantage ensued. In another condition, they were embedded in a series of musical stimuli. Here, a left ear advantage was found.[3] Clearly it is not the stimulus alone that determines the ear advantage. Two possible explanations exist. It could be that the context of speech versus music activates one hemisphere so that, by sheer momentum, that hemisphere dominates the identification.[4] Alternatively, it could be that the way the subject treats the stimulus determines to a large extent the hemisphere advantage. This effect of strategies is discussed below in more detail.

Artifacts in the Visual Half-Field Technique. Just as with the dichotic listening procedure, we should be sure we know how the subject treats the visual stimulus in question. As with the auditory test, both input strategies and processing strategies affect the lateral asymmetry. There may be a "right side of body" bias in right-handers, giving an advantage to the right visual field. More importantly, though, is the problem of attentional scanning—of paying attention in a left-to-right fashion due to the habit in reading. If words are presented horizontally, for example, one in each visual field, one would think that the closer the letter of a word is to the fixation point, the better it would be read. But this is not the case. As in shown in Figure 15.1, there is a left-to-right progression in accuracy even for the word in the left visual field. Thus, any study that uses words presented horizontally will have the scanning artifact to contend with, usually contributing to a right visual field advantage. This effect is, of course, independent of the left-sided dominance for speech. This artifact is a danger especially in studies

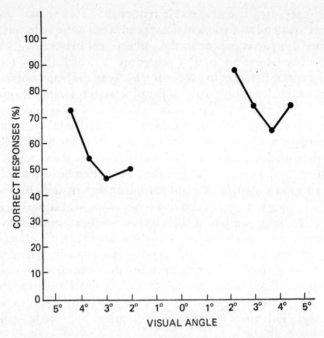

FIGURE 15.1. When words are presented horizontally in the visual half-field paradigm, the left-side word is more poorly read because the subject loses time in scanning it from left to right. From Segalowitz, S.J. 1979. Does bilateral word reading measure brain lateralization, differential information in the words, or attentional scanning? Paper presented at the American Psychological Association, New York, NY.

comparing good and poor readers. Since the activity of reading, which is required by the paradigm itself, is biased in favor of the right visual field, we would expect those with deviant reading patterns[5] to show less of this bias. When a lack of asymmetry is found only in the poor readers, it is tempting to conclude that these subjects are not lateralized, implying that this is the source of their problem rather than a manifestation of it!

Processing strategies—how subjects treat the task—are equally crucial in the visual paradigm as in the auditory. If two people look at the same stimulus but perform different activities with it, we should expect there to be different brain correlates for the task.

228

Returning again to the study of Ross and Turkewitz for illustration (see Chapter 6), some subjects treat face recognition as an analytic task, others as a holistic one. Naturally they produce different asymmetry scores.[6]

Coping with Artifacts. Both of the most popular experimental techniques, then, must be carefully used and interpreted. It is simply not the case that a behavioral difference invariably indicates brain lateralization, nor that a lack of one indicates no lateralization. Other factors can overshadow the rather fragile lateralization effects found with these techniques. Other procedures, such as lateral eye movements or bimanual tasks, can equally be affected by input strategies. The problem is that although we may be interested in hemispheric asymmetries in processing capabilities (is one hemisphere better than the other?), the very act of doing the task sets up attentional asymmetries that affect the resulting responses. Such attentional asymmetries are interesting, but possibly for reasons other than brain lateralization.

One response to the multiple problems with behavioral measures has been to develop nonbehavioral tasks, such as EEG and cerebral blood flow measures, so-called "direct measures" of brain activity. These avoid the artifacts of input biases because the subject does not have to struggle to get all the information. In these paradigms, there is no competition between ears or requirement for rapid reading of peripheral information. The stimuli can be presented comfortably. In many such experiments, the subject does nothing in particular, besides listen to or watch the stimuli. When asking questions about the processing of stimulus characteristics, such as the studies on speech discussed in Chapter 12, the paradigm is certainly free of the kinds of artifacts discussed earlier. But when the subject must do something with the input, such as remember it or solve some problem, the same strategy issues arise. There is no foolproof method for determining lateralization of functions in normals.

However, the variety of techniques that exist can be useful in their diversity. If several methods, each with different interpretation problems, agree on the results, we develop some confidence in the conclusion. Such convergence is not without interpretive problems. Remember that the direct measures reflect participation in the task, while dichotic listening and visual half-field procedures reflect dominance. But when they all agree, life is simpler.

Strategies and Individual Differences

It should be clear by now that many factors go into making an asymmetry score on a lateralization test: attentional biases, the physical characteristics of the stimulus, the subject's attitude towards the stimulus, and, of course, actual hemisphere asymmetries for the processing in question. The last two factors are clearly related. For example, Tom Bever and Robert Chiarello gave a variant on the dichotic listening procedure to musicians and nonmusicians. They presented a melody to one ear for comparison with subsequent melodies. Musically experienced subjects had a right ear advantage for recognition of the melodies whereas nonexperienced subjects showed a left ear advantage for this task. Does this mean that musicians and nonmusicians have differently organized brains? Not at all. Rather, the strategy the subject applied to the task was different for each group. Not surprisingly, the musically trained subjects were quite adept at analyzing a melody into its constituent parts (shown on another part of the task). Those without training use a more holistic strategy, favoring the right hemisphere. Given the nature of the task, an analytic strategy is much more appropriate in order to get correct answers. Consistent with this is the finding that the more correct items a subject gets, the greater the right ear advantage.[7] Thus the strategy a subject uses, dependent no doubt to a large extent on past experience, can determine the apparent lateralization for the task.

As discussed in more detail in Part III, there are a number of subject variables leading to variation in such apparent lateralization. A well-documented one is a sex difference in degree of asymmetry shown: When there are differences, it is the women who tend toward less asymmetry.[8] Again we are stuck with the vital question, Is this difference one in brain organization or only how the subject approaches the task? Cognitive style differences could be at the root of many or even all differences in lateralization between groups. Until recently, this difficulty in interpretation has not been considered critical. Having had experience with the difficulty, though, researchers must now attend to proper experimental control conditions to aid in interpretations.

Using Relative Measures

Interpreting a single lateralization measure is hazardous. Only Wada testing or studies of brain-damaged patients are unequivocal about asymmetrical representation. The problem with these methods, though, is that it is not clear *what* it is that is represented asymmetrically. The deficits are usually so global that it is impossible to speak of mechanisms.

So how can we avoid the confounding of input strategies, processing strategies, and true lateralization, a confounding that is necessary when we use a single laterality measure? The solution is to use *relative measures*. We can illustrate this with some data presented in Figure 15.2. We see here the results of two subjects, each tested six times over a period of three weeks on two visual half-field tasks, one verbal and one spatial. The verbal task involved reading vertically-presented nonsense syllables. Vertical presentation avoids the confounding of left-to-right attentional scanning; the use of nonsense syllables requires that the words be read phonically, since they cannot be recognized as whole words. The spatial task involved reading the times on a clock face that had no numbers, only marks to indicate the twelve divisions. In both cases, the subject responded verbally. Note that the two tasks had similar input and output requirements. Only the content of the stimulus, and therefore presumably the type of mental processing that went on, differed.[9] In Figure 15.2, we see the data plotted on a graph where the vertical axis represents the degree of asymmetry, positive being a left hemisphere superiority, negative a right-superiority, and zero no asymmetry. The two subjects here showed considerable variability over time, yet the pattern is consistent. The verbal stimuli produced a greater left-hemisphere advantage than the right. The pattern is consistent across the two subjects, despite the fact that one has a general right visual field advantage (her scores are all positive) and the other a general left visual field advantage (her scores are all negative). The multiple testing allows us to determine the reliability of the subject's scores. The relative measure—the relationship

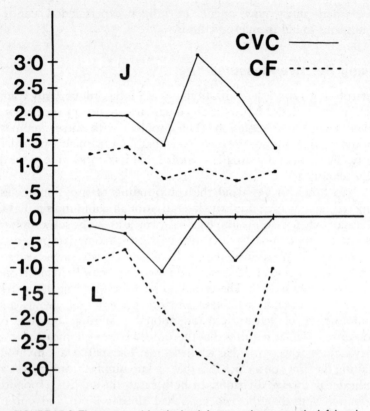

FIGURE 15.2. The more positive the lambda score, the greater the left hemisphere (right visual field) advantage for reading these nonsense syllable (CVC) and clockface (CF) stimuli. These two subjects were tested over 6 sessions. Both show a greater left hemisphere advantage for the verbal material, yet clearly one subject has an overall bias to one side, the other to the other side. Thus, while their *hemisphericity* may differ, their patterns of lateralization are the same. From Segalowitz & Orr (1981).

between the scores for the two lateralization tasks—allows us to control for the particular input processes that produce artifacts and any idiosyncracies the particular subject may have (such as a general visual field bias to one side). These are controlled because they hold for both measures and the subject acts as his or her own control.

With this research approach, it would be possible to examine differences between left- and right-handers without the problem of attentional biases. Similarly the issues of sex and cognitive style differences can be addressed without the main variable in question turning into an artifact. It should be noted, however, that the use of relative measures subtly changes the research question. Instead of asking whether or not a particular function is lateralized, we must talk about the *relative* asymmetry of a function. Thus, in the example given, the verbal task for both subjects involved more left-hemisphere advantage relative to the spatial task. This does not mean that "language is left" and "spatial is right." After all, in one subject, both verbal and spatial scores are positive and for the other, both are negative. Rather, for both language is more left-lateralized and the spatial function more right-sided. Making absolute statements on the basis of laterality measures as we have discussed simply ignores the relativity issue but does not solve it.

NOTES

1. Kimura (1961b). See Bryden (1978) for more detail on this point.
2. See Bryden (1978) and Gruber & Segalowitz (1977) for this and further points.
3. Spellacy & Blumstein (1970).
4. Kinsbourne (1972) argues in favor of this approach. See Chapter 4 for fuller discussion of the "momentum" model.
5. Pavlidis (1981).
6. Ross & Turkewitz (in press). See also Segalowitz & Stewart (1979) and Segalowitz & Bryden (in press) for further discussion on this point.
7. Bever & Chiarello (1974), Gordon (1975). Differences in lateralization effects between musicians and nonmusicians have been reported numerous times since Bever & Chiarello's report.
8. See Bryden (1979b) and Segalowitz & Bryden (in press).
9. Segalowitz & Orr (1981).

chapter sixteen

Mapping the mind onto the brain

The search for an understanding of the brain's activity is fraught with philosophical dilemmas as well as the need for data. Some of these problems have already been raised as empirical issues, such as deciding whether sex differences in lateralization are due to different choices of strategy or to biological differences. We can take this issue further, however. We can ask, whenever differences in hemisphere function are found whether they are due to biological or psychological factors. Implicit in much of the literature on brain lateralization (especially in the articles in the popular press) is the computer distinction that some organization is "hard-wired" and other is "soft-wired." Hard-wired structures cannot be changed except by physical alteration. Soft-wired structures are reprogrammable. They can be changed at will. Thus, in a computer, whether a program adds or subtracts two numbers is a soft-wiring (or software) issue. How the machine does so is a hard-wiring (or hardware) issue.

In humans, since some functions are more or less fixed compared to others, we consider there to be various levels of soft-wiring. When some brain organization is found at birth and stays relatively consistent throughout life, it is tempting to refer to this structure as hard-wired. In this category may fall some processes involved in the perception of speech. Many lateralization effects, however, are not due to the stimuli alone, but to the attitude or approach of the subject. In such cases, it seems appropriate to consider the effect of a soft-wiring one. If the software (i.e. strategies) can override hard-wiring effects, can we ever tell whether two groups differing in lateralization scores vary in biological or in psychological organization? When comparing groups, if we cannot differentiate the two types of effects, does the distinction still make sense?

This kind of problem is related to the debate on biological reductionism, basic to this whole enterprise: To what extent is it useful and appropriate to look for biological factors to help us understand and explain psychological facts? The debate has been long and, at times, acrimonious.[1] There are two aspects that concern us here. Can a study of the brain help us understand why it is that some people are different from others? And can we learn more about ourselves by examining the brain?

The first question applies to the issue of differences in talents across people: Does the higher linguistic skill of some people indicate that they have an inborn left hemisphere that is more efficient and perhaps more active as well, or could the differences in hemispheric function between them and less verbal people be accounted for simply by linguistic skill? In other words, which comes first, the biological difference or the psychological difference? This issue plays havoc with the hardware-software distinction. We are far from answering it, for although we know that there is a structural organization to the brain that develops before and after birth, we also know that some of this organization can be modified by experience.

The second aspect is even more contentious. Throughout this book, we have focused on links between brain function and psychological experience that are mutually reinforcing, that is, on research findings concerning behavior that give us insight about the organization of the brain, and conversely, brain organization data that may help us better understand our psychological theories. At some level of brain analysis, there can be useful links. At more detailed levels, though, the usefulness of the cross-talk breaks down. As Steven Rose has written,

> to study molecular neurobiology in order to understand brain and
> behavior is like studying the construction of a tape recorder and the
> composition of the magnetic tape in order to understand the music
> recorded on it.[2]

In the study of brain lateralization, we do not examine the molecular
level. However, we must be careful not to lose sight of the dangers
inherent in brain-mind mapping. For some questions, the proper
study of behavior may be only behavior itself.

Complementarity. Since the premise of the study of brain
lateralization is the dichotomy of left and right, it is natural to stress
the different strengths of each side of the brain. Implicit in this is the
notion that each side has its own strengths. Typically, this difference
has been characterized as verbal versus spatial thought, or analytic
versus holistic thinking. These dichotomies, however, have always
been based on group effects, the differences found in the average performance of a group of right and left hemispheres, so to speak. It has
not been demonstrated conclusively that in an individual brain, if
one hemisphere is specialized for verbal skills, the other is dominant
for spatial skills.[3] This needs to be examined, because much of our
understanding of hemispheric function lies in the balance. If one
hemisphere can be dominant for both sets of functions, what purpose
does the other one serve, keeping in mind that dominance and
competence are not synonymous? If the hemispheres do complement
each other, do they for all aspects of lateralization, dominance,
competence and participation? This principle of complementarity,
taken for granted for so long, should be investigated systematically.
Clearly, many of the issues discussed earlier concerning detecting
variation in brain lateralization among individuals are relevant here.

Causes and Effects. Related to the first aspect of the
biological reductionism issue—what is responsible for differences
between people—is the cause-effect question. Given that a certain
pattern of brain activity and a certain experience correspond to each
other, does the brain activity underlie the experience or is the
thinking responsible for the brain activity pattern? In other words, if
a person uses a certain strategy that reflects a neuropsychological
pattern, is the choice a biological or a psychological one? At present,

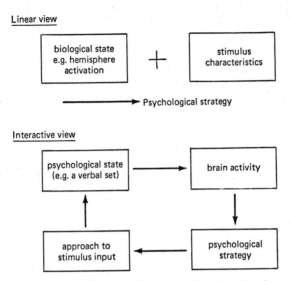

Linear view

| biological state e.g. hemisphere activation | $+$ | stimulus characteristics |

→ Psychological strategy

Interactive view

psychological state (e.g. a verbal set) → brain activity → psychological strategy → approach to stimulus input → psychological state (e.g. a verbal set)

FIGURE 16.1. The implicit models of mind-brain relationships involve the contrast between a linear system and an interactive system.

we have no way of knowing which aspect is more basic causally or whether it is always reasonable to ask such a question. In varying circumstances, each factor may accrue different weights. Biological factors are usually considered to be more basic than psychological ones, because it is the brain tissue that gives rise to the mind. Yet this relation need not apply to activity patterns. In Figure 16.1, we see the two models outlined. The contrast between the basic linear system and the interactive systems is familiar in many branches of the human and natural sciences.[4]

The Limits and Future of Brain Lateralization. The left-right distinction is only one of several we can make in discussing the organization of the brain. In a more detailed study of the brain, cortical-subcortical (up-down) and intrahemispheric (back-front, cross-lobe comparisons) distinctions play a more extensive role than the simple left-right one. There are severe limits to the usefulness of hemispheric asymmetries. Yet it is the most explored dimension. The reason is easy to see. Given the measures described throughout this book, many interesting studies can be done without the surgical training and facilities needed for "wet" physiology. The subsequent accessibility of brain-behavior study has broadened the acceptance of neurological issues in psychology in general.

The last decade's work on brain lateralization has changed our view of the human mind, and advanced our conceptualizing about how the brain operates. However, it has done this by simplifying the questions about brain-behavior relationships to a considerable extent. The simplification, however temporary, has been exceedingly useful in that more people now better appreciate the questions. Undoubtedly the next major advances in our understanding will involve complicating the situation to include some of the issues raised here.

NOTES

1. For example, the Soviets have long argued for a "materialist" behavioral science that rejects purely psychological constructs as idealist and bourgeois. See Rose & Rose (1973) for other political implications of reductionism.
2. Rose (1976). See also Rose & Rose (1973).
3. Unfortunately, clinical data are rarely presented in such a fashion as to clarify the matter. From Hécaen, DeAgostini & Monzon-Montes (1981), however, it is clear that in right handers, the incidence of disruption of spatial skills from right hemisphere damage compared to left hemisphere damage (a ratio of 2.5:1) is much smaller than the reverse for aphasia (5.7:1). One suspects, then, in the absence of a more direct study, that the two skills are not complementarily distributed.
4. For example, Dewey (1896) and Neisser (1976) present the interactive alternative to simpler information processing models of perception, and Kitchener (1978, 1980) and Lerner (1976, 1980) debate the nature of an interaction model in the biological and psychological development of the child.

Glossary

Agnosia An inability to recognize things that are otherwise well-known to the patient, often limited to a single sense modality.

Alpha The band of EEG wave patterns in the range of 8 to 13 cycles per second (Hz.), usually taken to indicate a lack of active thinking.

Anterior Referring to the forward parts of the brain.

Aphasia The loss of some language ability through brain damage.

Apraxia A disturbance in the performance of purposeful movements without paralysis, caused by brain damage.

ASL American Sign Language of the deaf, also referred to as Ameslan.

Averaged evoked response (AER) An average of many evoked responses to the same stimulus, thus cancelling out unrelated wave patterns.

Axon A (relatively) long extending arm of a neuron that propagates the electrical impulse from the cell body to other cells.

Beta Fast brain wave activity, above 13 cycles per second (Hz.), indicating active thinking.

Broca's aphasia A disturbance of language characterized by good comprehension but extremely halting, impaired production.

CBF Cerebral blood flow.

Cell body The core of the cell that contains the nucleus, in which resides the genetic material.

Cerebral commissures The bundles of fibers connecting homologous sites in the two hemispheres.

Cerebral cortex The surface grey matter of the cerebrum, considered responsible for higher cognitive functions.

Cerebrum The large, upper portion of the brain consisting of the left and right hemispheres.

Commissurotomy The cutting of the corpus callosum and possibly other cerebral commissures as well.

Complementarity The exclusive distribution of skills in the cerebral hemispheres, such that if language is represented in one hemisphere, some non-language skills are represented in the other.

Corpus callosum The largest of the commissures joining the two cerebral hemispheres.

Correlation coefficient A statistic used to reflect the degree of relation between two variables. A score of +1.0 indicates a positive relation, of -1.0 an inverse relation, and 0.0 no relation.

Cross-cueing In a split-brain patient, the giving of hints by one hemisphere to the other concerning information only transmitted to the former.

Dendrite An extension from the cell body of neurons that propagates electrical impulses to the cell body.

Dichhaptic task A task assessing hemisphere specialization by having the subject identify by touch two objects, one to each hand, presented simultaneously.

Dichotic listening A task designed to assess hemisphere specialization by sending simultaneous input to the two ears.

Dominant hemisphere The tendency for one hemisphere to control the processing of information in a particular task. Often used to refer to the hemisphere controlling speech.

Double dissociation The separation of two syndromes by finding the symptoms of one in the absence of the other and vice versa.

Dyslexia **A** disturbance in reading in the absence of other gross learning impairments.

EEG (electroencephalogram) **A** recording of brain wave patterns taken from electrodes placed on the scalp.

Embedded figures task A perceptual disembedding task that requires the subject to find a given figure in a complex scene.

Encoded speech Speech sounds that are not invariant acoustically in different speech contexts.

Evoked response The EEG response to a particular stimulus.

Facial agnosia See prosopagnosia.

Field dependence The tendency, when making a perceptual judgment, to be influenced by surrounding information.

Fluent aphasia See Wernicke's aphasia.

Frontal aphasia See Broca's aphasia.

Frontal lobe That portion of the cerebrum anterior to the Rolandic fissure.

Grey matter Cortical tissue consisting of cell bodies.

HAS The high amplitude sucking paradigm that allows babies some control on the stimulus input.

Hemispatial neglect The tendency for a patient with (almost always right hemisphere) brain damage to ignore one side of space. The side ignored is almost always the left side.

Hemisphericity The tendency for one hemisphere to be dominant independent of the task.

Holism A position in neuropsychology that treats the brain as a whole in its intellectual functioning.

Homologous Referring to the corresponding site in the other hemisphere.

Illicutionary force The pragmatic import of an utterance despite its grammatical form. Thus a demand is sometimes phrased as a question.

Isolation syndrome A rare syndrome of brain damage where the patient's language areas are intact, yet isolated from the rest of the cortex.

Kana The Japanese writing system involving syllabic units.

Kanji The Japanese writing system involving ideograms.

Localizationism A position in neuropsychology that represents the attempt to specify centers in the brain for psychological functions.

Millisecond One thousandth of a second.

Motor aphasia See Broca's aphasia.

Myelin The white cells that form a sheath around some nerve cells, and aid in the transmission of electrical impulses.

Neglect syndrome See hemispatial neglect.

Neuron A brain or nerve cell that is specialized as a conductor of impulses.

Nondominant hemisphere The hemisphere not dominant for speech.

Occipital lobe The rear portion of the cerebrum.

Parietal lobe The uppor portion of the cerebrum, posterior to the Rolandic fissure and above the temporal and occipital lobes.

Perseveration The involuntary repetition of an action.

Phoneme The abstract unit used in a language to represent a particular speech sound.

Phonology The study of and system of speech sounds in a language.

Phrenology The theory that specific faculties of mind are represented in specific places in the brain, and that the strength of these faculties in an individual can be ascertained by examining the skull, the shape of which is deemed to be affected by the growth of the faculties directly beneath.

Pineal gland A small brain structure which is not duplicated in each hemisphere, and therefore chosen by Descartes as the site of integration of the body and soul.

Plasticity The ability of the brain to recover functions lost through damage by reorganization.

Posterior Referring to the rear position of the brain.

Prosopagnosia (facial agnosia) An inability to recognize familiar faces.

Psychic blindness The loss of the ability to recognize objects despite intact vision.

Semantics The meanings of words and of their combinations and the rules governing those meanings.

Sinistrality Left-handedness.

Sodium Amytal The drug used in the Wada test.

Sprouting The regrowth of a cell's dendrites and axoms after damage.

Sylvian fissure A major crevice on the cerebrum separating the temporal and parietal lobes.

Syntax The system of rules in a language governing the ordering of words and the conjugation of words (morphology). Often referred to as grammar.

Temporal lobe The portion of the cerebrum below the Sylvian fissure.

Triangulation The use of more than one investigative technique to examine a phenomenon.

Visual half-field A field of vision to one side of the point of fixation.

Voice onset time The amount of time it takes for the vocal chords to start vibrating after the release of air in stop consonants (e.g. *b, g, p, k*).

Wada test A test given to neurological patients presurgically to determine the effects, primarily on speech, of the loss of one hemisphere. A barbituate, sodium amobarbitol (sodium amytal) is injected into the artery leading to one hemisphere.

Wernicke's aphasia A disturbance of language characterized by poor comprehension and fluent production, but with many word and sound substitutions.

White matter Connective fibers of brain cells consisting primarily of axons and their myelin coating.

References

Ades, A.E. 1974. Bilateral component in speech perception? *Journal of the Acoustical Society of America, 56,* 610–16.

Aitkin, L.M. & Webster, W.R. 1972. Medial geniculate body of the cat: organization and responses to tonal stimuli of neurons in ventral division. *Journal of Neurophysiology, 35,* 365–80.

Alajouanine, T. 1948. Aphasia and artistic realization. *Brain, 71,* 229–41.

Albert, M.L. & Baer, D. 1974. Time to understand. *Brain, 97,* 373–84.

Albert, M. & Obler, L. 1978. *The Bilingual Brain.* New York: Academic Press.

Albert, M.L., Sparks, R.W. & Helm, N.A. 1973. Melodic intonation therapy for aphasia. *Archives of Neurology, 29,* 130–31.

Allard, F. 1980. Sex, Space, and Sport. University of Waterloo, Department of Psychology.

Andreae, J.H. 1978. Descriptive and prescriptive names: commentary on the command neuron concept. *The Behavioral and Brain Sciences, 1,* 11–12.

Andrews, R.J. 1977. Aspects of language lateralization correlated with familial handedness. *Neuropsychologia, 15,* 769–78.

Annett, M. 1970. A classification of hand preference by association analysis. *British Journal of Psychology, 61,* 303-21.

Annett, M. 1972. The distribution of manual asymmetry. *British Journal of Psychology, 63,* 343-58.

Arndt, S. & Berger, D. 1978. Cognitive mode and asymmetry in cerebral functioning. *Cortex, 14,* 78-87.

Assal, G. 1973. Aphasie de Wernicke sans amusie chez un pianiste. *Revue Neurologique, 129,* 251-55.

Austin, J.L. 1962. *How To Do Things with Words.* New York: Oxford University Press.

Bakan, P. 1969. Hypnotizability, laterality of eye-movements and functional brain asymmetry. *Perceptual and Motor Skills, 28,* 927-32.

Bakan, P. 1971. Handedness and birth order. *Nature, 229,* 195.

Bakan, P. 1977. Left handedness and birth order revisited. *Neuropsychologia, 15,* 837-39.

Bakan, P. 1978. Dreaming, REM sleep, and the right hemisphere: a theoretical integration. *Journal of Altered States of Consciousness, 3,* 285-307.

Barerra, M.E., Dalrymple, A. & Witelson, S.F. 1978. Behavioral evidence of right hemisphere asymmetry in early infancy. Paper presented to the Canadian Psychological Association, Ottawa, Ontario.

Barsley, M. 1970. *Left-Handed Man in a Right-Handed World.* London: Pitman.

Benson, D.F. 1979. Aphasia. In Heilman & Valenstein (1979).

Benton, A.L. 1977. Historical notes on hemispheric dominance. *Archives of Neurology, 34,* 127-29.

Benton, A. 1979. Visuoperceptive, visuospatial, and visuoconstructive disorders. In Heilman & Valenstein (1979).

Berent, S. & Silverman, A.J. 1973. Field dependence and differences between visual and verbal learning tasks *Perceptual and Motor Skills, 36,* 1327-30.

Berlin, C.I. & Cullen, J.K. Jr. 1977. Acoustic problems in dichotic listening tasks. In Segalowitz & Gruber (1977a).

Berlin, C.I., Hughes, L.F. Lowe-Bell, S.S. & Berlin, H.L. 1973. Dichotic right ear advantage in children 5 to 13. *Cortex, 9,* 393-401.

Berlin, C.I. & McNeil, M.R. 1976. Dichotic Listening. In N.J. Lass (ed.) *Contemporary Issues in Experimental Phonetics.* Springfield, IL: C.C. Thomas.

Berlucchi, G., Brizzolara, D., Marzi, C., Rizzolatti, G. & Umilta, C. 1979. The role of stimulus discriminability and verbal codability in hemispheric specialization for visuospatial tasks. *Neuropsychologia, 17,* 195–202.

Bernstein, L. 1976. *The Unanswered Question.* Cambridge: Harvard University Press.

Bever, T.G. & Chiarello, R.J. 1974. Cerebral dominance in musicians and nonmusicians. *Science, 185,* 537–39.

Bever, T.G., Hurtig, R.R. & Handel, A.B. 1976. Analytic processing elicits right ear superiority in monaurally presented speech. *Neuropsychologia, 14,* 175–81.

Blackstock, E.G. 1978. Cerebral asymmetry and the development of early infantile autism. *Journal of Autism and Childhood Schizophrenia, 8,* 339–53.

Blakemore, C. 1970. Binocular depth perception and the optic chiasm. *Vision Research, 10,* 43–47.

Blumstein, S.E. 1981. Neurolinguistic disorders: language-brain relationships. In S.B. Filskov & T.J. Boll (eds.) *Handbook of Clinical Neuropsychology.* New York: John Wiley & Sons.

Blumstein, S. & Cooper, W.E. 1974. Hemispheric processing of intonation contours. *Cortex, 10,* 146–58.

Blumstein, S., Goodglass, H. & Tartter, V. 1975. The reliability of ear advantage in dichotic listening. *Brain and Language, 2,* 226–36.

Bogen, J. 1969. The other side of the brain: the appositional mind. *Bulletin of the Los Angeles Neurological Societies, 34,* 135–62.

Bogen, J.E. 1977. Some educational implications of hemispheric specialization. In McWittrock (ed.) *The Human Brain,* Englewood Cliffs: Prentice-Hall.

Bogen, J. 1979. The callosal syndrome. In Heilman & Valenstein (1979).

Bogen, J.E. & Bogen, G.M. 1969. The other side of the brain III: the corpus callosum and creativity, *Bulletin of the Los Angeles Neurological Societies, 34,* 191–217.

Bogen, J.E. & Gordon, H.W. 1971. Musical tests for functional lateralization with intracarotid amobarbital. *Nature, 230,* 524–25.

Borowy, T. & Goebel, R. 1976. Cerebral lateralization of speech: the effects of age, sex, race, and socioeconomic class. *Neuropsychologia, 14,* 363–70.

Bower, T.G.R. 1977. *A Primer of Infant Development.* San Francisco: Freeman.

Bowers, K. 1974. Hypnosis for the Seriously Curious. San Francisco: Brooks/Cole.

Bradshaw, J.L. 1980. Right-hemisphere language: familial and non-familial sinistrals, cognitive deficits and writing hand position in sinistrals, and concrete-abstract, imageable-nonimageable dimensions in word recognition. A review of interrelated issues. *Brain and Language, 10,* 172–88.

Bradshaw, J.L. & Taylor, M.J. 1979. A word-naming deficit in non-familial sinistrals? Laterality effects of vocal responses to tachistoscopically presented letter strings. *Neuropsychologia, 17,* 21–32.

Brann, A.W. & Myers, R.E. 1975. Central nervous system findings in the newborn monkey following severe in utero partial asphyxia. *Neurology, 25,* 327–38.

Bresson, F., Maury, L., Pierant-Le Bonniec, G. & de Schonen, S. 1977. Organization and lateralization of reaching in infants: an instance of asymmetric functions in hands colloboration. *Neuropsychologia, 15,* 311–20.

Brinkman, J. & Kuypers, H.G.J.M. 1972. Splitbrain monkeys: cerebral control of ipsilateral and contralateral arm, hand, and finger movements. *Science, 176,* 536–39.

Brown, W.S., Marsh, J.T. & Smith, J.C. 1973. Contextual meaning effects on speech-evoked potentials. *Behavioral Biology, 9,* 755–61.

Brown, W.S., Marsh, J.T. & Smith, J.C. 1976. Evoked potential waveform differences produced by the perception of different meanings of an ambiguous phrase. *Electroencephalograph and Clinical Neurophysiology, 41,* 113–23.

Bruder, G.E. & Yozawitz, A. 1979. Central auditory processing and lateralization in psychiatric patients. In Gruzelier & Flor-Henry (1979).

Bryden, M.P. 1965. Tachistoscopic recognition, handedness, and cerebral dominance. *Neuropsychologia, 3,* 1–8.

Bryden, M.P. 1970. Laterality effects in dichotic listening: relations with handedness and reading ability in children. *Neuropsychologia, 8,* 443–50.

Bryden, M.P. 1976. Response bias and hemispheric differences in dot localization. *Perception & Psychophysics, 9,* 23–28.

Bryden, M.P. 1978. Strategy effects in the assessment of hemispheric asymmetry. In G. Underwood (ed.) *Strategies of Information Processing.* London: Academic Press.

Bryden, M.P. 1979a. Possible genetic mechanisms of handedness and laterality. Paper presented at the Canadian Psychological Association meeting, Quebec, Quebec.

Bryden, M.P. 1979b. Evidence for sex-related differences in cerebral organization. In M. Wittig & A.C. Peterson (eds.) *Sex-Related Differences in Cognitive Functioning.* New York: Academic Press.

Bryden, M.P. (1982). *Laterality: Functional Asymmetry in the Intact Brain.* New York: Academic Press.

Bryden, M.P., Ley, R.G. & Sugarman, J.H. 1982. A left-ear advantage for identifying the emotional quality of tonal sequences. *Neuropsychologia, 20,* 83–87.

Buchsbaum, M. & Fedio, P. 1969. Visual information and evoked responses from the left and right hemispheres. *Electroencephalography and Clinical Neurophysiology, 26,* 266–72.

Buffrey, A.W.H. & Gray, J.A. 1972. Sex differences in the development of spatial and linguistic skills. In C. Ounsted & D.C. Taylor (eds.) *Gender Differences: Their Ontogeny and Significance.* London: Churchill Livingstone.

Cain, D.P. & Wada, J.A. 1979. An anatomical asymmetry in the baboon brain. *Brain, Behavior and Evolution, 16,* 222–26.

Cameron, R.F., Currier, R.D., & Haerer, A.F. 1971. Aphasia and literacy. *British Journal of Disorders of Communication, 6,* 161–63.

Capitani, E., Scotti, G. & Spinnler, H. 1978. Colour imperception in patients with focal excisions of the cerebral hemispheres. *Neuropsychologia, 16,* 491–96.

Caplan, P. & Kinsbourne, M. 1976. Baby drops the rattle: asymmetry of duration of grasp by infants. *Child Development, 47,* 532–34.

Capra, F. 1975. *The Tao of Physics.* Berkeley, CA: Shambhala.

Caramazza, A., Gordon, J., Zurif, E.B. & DeLuca, D. 1976. Right-hemispheric damage and verbal problem solving behavior. *Brain and Language, 3,* 41–46.

Carmon, A. & Gombos, G.M. 1970. A physiological vascular correlate of hand preference: possible implications with respect to hemispheric cerebral dominance. *Neuropsychologia, 8,* 119–28.

Carmon, A., Lavy, S., Gordon, H. & Portnoy, Z. 1975. Hemispheric differences in CBF during verbal and nonverbal tasks. *Brain Work, 8,* 414–23.

Carmon, A. & Nachshon, I. 1973. Ear asymmetry in perception of emotional non-verbal stimuli. *Acta Psychologica, 37,* 351–57.

Chapman, R.M., Bragdon, H.R., Chapman, J.A. & McCrary, J.W. 1977. Semantic meaning of words and averaged evoked potentials. In J.E. Desmedt (ed.) *Recent Developments in the Psychobiology of Language: The Cerebral Evoked Potential Approach.* London: Oxford University Press.

Clarke, E. & Dewhurst, K. 1972. *An Illustrated History of Brain Function.* Berkeley: University of California Press.

Cohen, B.D., Berent, S. & Silverman, A.J. 1973. Field-dependence and lateralization of function in the human brain. *Archives of General Psychiatry, 28,* 165–67.

Cohen, G. 1972. Hemispheric differences in serial versus parallel processing. *Journal of Experimental Psychology, 97,* 349–56.

Cohen, R.A. 1969. Conceptual styles, culture conflict, and nonverbal tests of intelligence. *American Anthropologist, 71,* 828–56.

Colby, K.M. & Parkinson, C. 1977. Handedness in autistic children. *Journal of Autism and Childhood Schizophrenia, 7,* 3–9.

Collins, R.L. 1977. Toward an admissable genetic model for the inheritance of the degree and direction of asymmetry. In Harnad, Doty, Goldstein, Jaynes & Krauthamer (1977).

Cometa, M.S. & Eson, M.E. 1978. Logical operations and metaphor in interpreting a Piagetian model. *Child Development, 49,* 649–59.

Corballis, M.C. & Beale, I.L. 1976. *The Psychology of Left and Right.* Hillsdale, NJ: Lawrence Erlbaum Associates.

Corballis, M.C. & Morgan, M.J. 1978. On the biological basis of human laterality: I. Evidence for a maturational left-right gradient. *The Behavioral and Brain Sciences, 2,* 261-69.

Coren, S. & Porac, C. 1977. Fifty centuries of right-handedness: the historical record. *Science, 198,* 631-32.

Coren, S., Porac, C. & Duncan, P. (1981). Lateral preference behaviors in pre-school children and young children. *Child Development, 52,* 443-50.

Crovitz, H.F. & Zener, K. 1962. A group test for assessing hand and eye dominance. *American Journal of Psychology, 75,* 271-76.

Crowne, D., Yeo, C.H. & Russell, I.S. 1981. The effects of unilateral frontal eye field lesions in the monkey: visual motor guidance and avoidance behavior. *Behavioral Brain Research, 2,* 165-87.

Curry, F. 1968. A comparison of the performances of a right hemispherectomized subject and 25 normals on four dichotic listening tasks. *Cortex, 4,* 144-53.

Curtiss, S. 1977. *Genie.* New York: Academic Press.

Cutting, J.E. 1974. Two left-hemisphere mechanisms in speech perception. *Perception & Psychophysics, 16,* 601-12.

Dabbs, J.M. 1980. Left-right differences in cerebral blood flow and cognition. *Psychophysiology, 17,* 548-51.

Dabbs, J.M. & Choo, G. 1980. Left-right carotid blood flow predicts specialized mental ability. *Neuropsychologia, 18,* 711-13.

Damasio, A.R., Castro-Caldas, A., Grosso, J.T. & Ferro, J.M. 1976. Brain specialization for language does not depend on literacy. *Archives of Neurology, 33,* 300-01.

Damasio, A.R. & Maurer, R.G. 1978. A neurological model for childhood autism. *Archives of Neurology, 35,* 77-786.

Danly, M., Cooper, W.E. & Shapiro, B. in press. Fundamental frequency, language processing, and linguistic structure in Wernicke's aphasia. *Brain and Language.*

Danly, M. & Shapiro, B. 1982. Speech prosody in Broca's aphasia. *Brain and Language, 16,* 171-90.

Darwin, C.J. 1971. Ear differences in the recall of fricatives and vowels. *Quarterly Journal of Experimental Psychology, 23,* 46-62.

Darwin, C.J. 1974. Ear differences and hemispheric specialization. In F.O. Schmitt & F.G. Warden (eds.) *Neurosciences: Third Study Program*. Cambridge: MIT Press.

Davidoff, J. 1977. Hemispheric differences in dot detection. *Cortex, 13*, 434–44.

Davidson, R.J. & Schwartz, G.E. 1977. The influence of musical training on patterns of EEG asymmetry during musical and non-musical self-generation tasks. *Psychophysiology, 14*, 58–63.

Dawson, G. 1981. Hemisphere functioning in autistic individuals. Paper presented at the International Neuropsychological Society, Atlanta, Georgia.

Dawson, G., Warrenburg, S. & Fuller, P. 1982. Cerebral lateralization in individuals diagnosed as autistic in early childhood. *Brain and Language, 15*, 353–68.

Dawson, J.L.M.B. 1977. An anthropological perspective on the evolution and lateralization of the brain. *Annals of the New York Academy of Sciences, 299*, 427–47.

Debes, J.L. 1977. Visuocultural influences on lateralization. *Annals of the New York Academy of Sciences, 299*, 474–76.

Dee, H. & Fontenot, D. 1973. Cerebral dominance and lateral differences in perception and memory. *Neuropsychologia, 11*, 167–73.

Dennenberg, V.H., Garbanati, J., Sherman, G., Yutzey, D.A. & Kaplan, R. 1978. Infantile stimulation induces brain lateralization in rats. *Science, 201*, 1150–52.

Dennis, M. 1976. Impaired sensory and motor differentiation with corpus callosum agenesis: a lack of callosal inhibition during ontogeny? *Neuropsychologia, 14*, 455–69.

Dennis, M. 1979. Language acquisition in a single hemisphere: semantic organization. In D. Caplan (ed.) *Biological Studies of Mental Processes*. Cambridge: MIT Press.

Dennis, M., Lovett, M. & Wiegel-Crump, C.A. 1981. Written language acquisition after left or right hemidecortication in infancy. *Brain and Language, 12*, 54–91.

Dennis, M. & Whitaker, H.A. 1976. Language acquisition following hemidecortication: linguistic superiority of the left over the right hemisphere. *Brain and Language, 3*, 404–33.

Dennis, M. & Whitaker, H.A. 1977. Hemispheric equipotentiality and language acquisition. In Segalowitz & Gruber (1977a).

Dewey, J. 1896. The reflex arc concept in psychology. *Psychological Review, 3,* 357-70.

Dewson, J.H. III 1977. Preliminary evidence of hemispheric asymmetry of auditory function in monkeys. In Harnad, Doty, Goldstein, Jaynes & Krauthamer (1977).

Dimond, S.J. 1979. Disconnection and psychopathology. In Gruzelier & Flor-Henry (1979).

Dimond, S.J., Scammell, R., Pryce, I.J., Huws, D. & Gray, C. 1980. Some failures of intermanual and cross-lateral transfer in chronic schizophrenia. *Journal of Abnormal Psychology, 89,* 505-09.

Dingwall, W.O. & Whitaker, H.A. 1974. Neurolinguistics. *Annual Review of Anthropology, 3,* 323-56.

Dirkes, M.A. 1978. The role of divergent production in the learning process. *American Psychologist, 33,* 815-20.

Doehring, D. 1979. Statistical classification of children with reading problems. *Journal of Clinical Neuropsychology, 1,* 5-16.

Dorman, M.F. & Geffner, D.S. 1974. Hemispheric specialization for speech perception in six-year-old black and white children from low and middle socioeconomic classes. *Cortex, 10,* 171-76.

Dumas, R. & Morgan, A. 1975. EEG asymmetry as a function of occupation, task, and task difficulty. *Neuropsychologia, 13,* 219-28.

Efron, R. 1963. Temporal perception, aphasia and déja vù. *Brain, 86,* 403-24.

Ehrlichman, H. & Weinberger, A. 1978. Lateral eye movements and hemispheric asymmetry: a critical review. *Psychological Bulletin, 85,* 1080-1111.

Eimas, P.D., Siqueland, F.R., Juscyk, P. & Vigorito, J. 1971. Speech perception in infants. *Science, 171,* 303-06.

Entus, A.K. 1977. Hemispheric asymmetry in processing of dichotically presented speech and nonspeech stimuli by infants. In Segalowitz & Gruber (1977a).

Erikson, E.H. 1963. *Childhood and Society.* New York: W.W. Norton.

Evans, F.J. 1979. Hypnosis and sleep: techniques for exploring cognitive activity during sleep. In E. Fromm & R.E. Shor (eds.) *Hypnosis: Developments in Research and New Perspectives,* second edition. New York: Aldine.

Evans, G.W. 1980. Environmental cognition. *Psychological Bulletin, 88,* 259-87.

Fennell, E.B., Bowers, D. & Satz, P. 1977. Within-modal and cross-modal reliabilities of two laterality tests. *Brain and Language, 4,* 63-69.

Fischer, F.W., Liberman, I.Y. & Shankweiler, D. 1978. Reading reversals and developmental dyslexia: a further study. *Cortex, 14,* 496-510.

Flor-Henry, P. 1976. Lateralized temporal-limbic dysfunction and psychopathology. *Annals of the New York Academy of Sciences, 280,* 777-95.

Flor-Henry, P. 1979. Commentary on theoretical issues and neuro-psychological and electroencephalographic findings. In Gruzelier & Flor-Henry (1979).

Foldi, N.S., Cicone, M. & Gardner, H. (1983). Pragmatic aspects of communication in brain damaged patients. In Segalowitz (1983).

Frisch, H.L. 1977. Sex stereotypes in adult-infant play. *Child Development, 48,* 1671-75.

Frumkin, L.R., Ripley, H.S. & Cox, G.B. 1978. Changes in cerebral hemispheric lateralization with hypnosis. *Biological Psychiatry, 13,* 741-50.

Gainotti, G. 1969. Réactions "catastrophiques" et manifestations l'indifference au cours des atteintes cérébrales. *Neuropsychologia, 7,* 195-204.

Gainotti, G. 1972. Emotional behavior and hemispheric side of the lesion. *Cortex, 8,* 41-55.

Galaburda, A.M., Lemay, M., Kemper, T.L. & Geschwind, N. 1978. Right-left asymmetries in the brain. *Science, 199,* 852-56.

Galin, D. 1974. Implications for psychiatry of left and right cerebral specialization. *Archives of General Psychiatry, 31,* 572-83.

Galin, D. 1976. The two modes of consciousness and the two halves of the brain. In P.R. Lee, R.E. Ornstein, D. Galin, A. Deikman & C.T. Tart (eds.) *Symposium on Consciousness.* New York· Viking Press.

Galin, D. 1978. Effects of task difficulty on EEG measures of cerebral engagement. *Neuropsychologia, 16*, 461-72.

Galin, D. 1979. EEG asymmetries in right and left hemispheres. Presented at the American Psychological Association, New York.

Galin, Diamond R. & Branff, D. 1977. Lateralization of conversion symptoms: more frequent on the left. *American Journal of Psychiatry, 134*, 578-80.

Galin, D., Johnstone, J., Nakell, L. & Herron, J. 1979. Development of the capacity for tactile information transfer between hemispheres in normal children. *Science, 204*, 1330-32.

Galin, D. & Ornstein, R. 1972. Lateral specialization of cognitive mode: an EEG study. *Psychophysiology, 9*, 412-18.

Galin, D. & Ornstein, R. 1974. Individual differences in cognitive style—I. Reflective eye movements. *Neuropsychologia, 12*, 367-76.

Gardner, H. 1974. *The Shattered Mind*. New York: Vintage Books.

Gardner, H., Ling, P.K., Flamm, L. & Silverman, J. 1975. Comprehension and appreciation of humor in brain-damaged patients. *Brain, 98*, 399-412.

Gardner, H., Silverman, J., Wapner, W. & Zurif, E. 1978. The appreciation of antonymic contrasts in aphasia. *Brain and Language, 6*, 301-17.

Gardiner, M.F. & Walter, D.O. 1977. Evidence of hemispheric specialization from infant EEG.

Gazzaniga, M.S. 1970. *The Bisected Brain*. New York: Appelton-Century-Crofts.

Gazzaniga, M.S. & Hillyard, S.A. 1971. Language and speech capacity of the right hemisphere. *Neuropsychologia, 9*, 273-80.

Gazzaniga, M.S. & LeDoux, J.E. 1978. *The Integrated Mind*. New York: Plenum Press.

Geffner, D.S. & Dorman, M.F. 1976. Hemispheric specialization for speech perception in four-year-old children from low and middle socio-economic classes. *Cortex, 12*, 71-73.

Geffner, D. & Hochberg, I. 1971. Ear laterality performance from low and middle socioeconomic levels on a verbal dichotic listening task. *Cortex, 7*, 193-203.

Geschwind, N. 1965. Disconnexion syndromes in animals and man. *Brain, 88*, 237-94.

Geschwind, N. 1972. Language and the brain. *Scientific American,* *226,* 76–83.

Geschwind, N. & Levitsky, W. 1968. Human brain: left-right asymmetries in temporal speech region. *Speech, 161,* 186–87.

Geschwind, N. Quadfasel, F.A. & Segarra, J.M. 1968. Isolation of the speech area. *Neuropsychologia, 6,* 327–40.

Gesell, A. & Ames, L. 1947. The development of handedness. *Journal of Genetic Psychology, 70,* 155–75.

Giannitrapani, D. 1967. Developing concepts of lateralization of cerebral functions. *Cortex, 3,* 353–70.

Gilbert, C. 1977. Non-verbal perceptual abilities in relation to left-handedness and cerebral lateralization. *Neuropsychologia, 15,* 779–91.

Glanville, B.B., Best, C.T. & Levenson, R. 1977. A cardiac measure of cerebral asymmetries in infant auditory perception. *Developmental Psychology, 13,* 54–59.

Glassman, R.B. 1978. The logic of the lesion experiment and its role in the neural sciences. In S. Finger (ed.) *Recovery From Brain Damage: Research and Theory.* New York: Plenum.

Godfrey, J. 1974. Perceptual difficulty and the right ear advantage for vowels. *Brain and Language, 1,* 323–35.

Goldman, P.S. & Brown, R.M. 1975. The influence of neonatal androgen on the development of cortical function in the rhesus monkey. *Society for Neuroscience Abstracts, 1,* 494.

Goldman, P.S., Crawford, H.T., Stokes, L.P., Galkin, T.W. & Rosvold, H.E. 1974. Sex-dependent behavioral effects of cerebral cortical lesions in the developing rhesus monkey. *Science, 186,* 540–42.

Goldstein, K. & Blackman, S. 1978. *Cognitive Style.* New York: Wiley.

Goodglass, H. 1976. Agrammatism. In H. Whitaker & H.A. Whitaker (eds.) *Studies in Neurolinguistics, Vol. 1.* New York: Academic Press.

Goodglass, H. & Geschwind, N. 1976. Language disorders (aphasia). In E.C. Carterette & M.P. Friedman (eds.) *Handbook of Perception, Vol. 8: Language and Speech.* New York: Academic Press.

Goodglass, H. & Kaplan, E. 1972. *The Assessment of Aphasia and Related Disorders.* Philadelphia: Lea & Febiger.

Gordon, H.W. 1975. Hemispheric asymmetry and musical performance. *Science, 189,* 68–69.

Gordon, H.W. 1980. Cognitive asymmetry in dyslexic families. *Neuropsychologia, 18,* 645–56.

Gordon, H.W., Frooman, B. & Lavie, P. 1982. Shift in cognitive asymmetries between wakings from REM and NREM sleep. *Neuropsychologia, 20,* 99–103.

Gott, P.S. & Saul, R.E. 1978. Agenesis of the corpus callosum: limits of functional compensation. *Neurology, 28,* 1272–79.

Greenough, W.T. 1975. Experiental modification of the developing brain. *American Scientist, 63,* 37–46.

Greenwood, P., Wilson, D.H. & Gazzaniga, M.S. 1977. Dream report following commissurotomy. *Cortex, 13,* 311–16.

Grossman, M. & Carey, S. 1978. Word-learning after brain damage. Presented at Academy of Aphasia, Chicago.

Gruber, F.A. & Segalowitz, S.J. 1977. Some issues and methods in the neuropsychology of language. In Segalowitz & Gruber (1977a).

Gruzelier, J. 1979. Synthesis and critical review of the evidence for hemisphere asymmetries of function in psychopathology. In Gruzelier & Flor-Henry (1979).

Gruzelier, J. & Flor-Henry, P. 1979. *Hemisphere Asymmetries of Function in Psychopathology.* Amsterdam: Elsevier/North Holland.

Gur, R.C. & Gur, R.E. 1974. Handedness, sex, and eyedness as moderating variables in the relation between hypnotic susceptibility and functional brain asymmetry. *Journal of Abnormal Psychology, 83,* 635–43.

Gur, R.E. 1978. Left hemisphere dysfunction and left hemisphere overactivation in schizophrenia. *Journal of Abnormal Psychology, 87,* 226–38.

Gur, R.E. 1979. Hemispheric overactivation in schizophrenia. In J. Gruzelier & P. Flor-Henry (eds). *Hemisphere Asymmetries of Function in Psychopathology.* Amsterdam: Elsevier/North-Holland.

Gur, R.E., Gur, R.C. & Marshalek, B. 1975. Classroom seating and functional brain asymmetry. *Journal of Educational Psychology, 67,* 151–53.

Hall, J.L. II & Goldstein, M.H. Jr. 1968. Representation of binaural stimuli by single units in primary auditory cortex of unanesthetized cats. *Journal of the Acoustical Society of America, 43,* 456-61.

Halverson, H. 1937a, b. Studies of the grasping responses of early infancy, I & II. *Journal of Genetic Psychology, 51,* 371-92 and 393-424.

Hamilton, C.R. 1977. An assessment of hemispheric specialization in monkeys. *Annals of the New York Academy of Sciences, 299,* 222-32.

Hammond, G.R. 1982. Hemispheric differences in temporal resolution. *Brain and Cognition, 1,* 95-118.

Hardyck, C. & Haapanen, R. 1979. Educating both halves of the brain: educational breakthrough or neuromythology? *Journal of School Psychology, 17,* 219-30.

Hardyck, C. & Petrinovitch, F. 1977. Left-handedness. *Psychological Bulletin, 84,* 385-404.

Hardyck, C., Petrinovitch, L.F. & Goldman, R.D. 1976. Left-handedness and cognitive deficit. *Cortex, 12,* 266-79.

Harnard, S.R., Doty, R.W., Goldstein, L., Jaynes, J. & Krauthamer, G. (eds.) 1977. *Lateralization in the Nervous System.* New York: Academic Press.

Harnad, S.R., Steklis, H.D. & Lancaster, J. (eds.) 1976. *Origins and Evolution of Language and Speech. Annals of the New York Academy of Sciences, 280.*

Harris, A.J. 1958. *Harris Tests of Lateral Dominance,* third edition. New York: The Psychological Corporation.

Harris, L.J. 1978. Sex differences in spatial ability: possible environmental, genetic, and neurological factors. In M. Kinsbourne (ed.) *Asymmetrical Function of the Brain.* Cambridge: Cambridge University Press.

Harris, L.J. 1980. Left-handedness: early theories, facts, and fancies. In Herron (1980).

Harshman, R.A., Remington, R. & Krashen, S.D. 1975. Sex, language, and the brain, Part II: Evidence from dichotic listening for adult sex differences in verbal lateralization. Unpublished manuscript, University of California, Los Angeles.

Hatta, T. 1977. Recognition of Japanese *Kanji* in the left and right visual fields. *Neuropsychologia, 15,* 685-88.

Hécaen, H. & Ajuriaguerra, J. 1964. *Left-Handedness and Cerebral Dominance*. New York: Grune & Stratton.

Hécaen, H. & Albert, M.L. 1978. *Human Neuropsychology*. New York: Wiley.

Hécaen, H., DeAgostini, M. & Monzon-Montes, A. 1981. Cerebral organization in left-handers. *Brain and Language, 12*, 261-84.

Hécaen, H. & Sauget, J. 1971. Cerebral dominance in left-handed subjects. *Cortex, 7*, 19-48.

Heeschen, C. & Jürgens, R. 1977. Pragmatic-semantic and syntactic factors influencing ear differences in dichotic listening. *Cortex, 13*, 74-84.

Heilman, K.M., Rothi, L., Campanella, D. & Wolfson, S. 1979. Wernicke's and global aphasia without alexia. *Archives of Neurology, 36*, 129-33.

Heilman, K.M., Scholes, R. & Watson, R.T. 1975. Auditory affective agnosia: disturbed comprehension of affective speech. *Journal of Neurology, Neurosurgery, and Psychiatry, 38*, 69-72.

Heilman, K.M. & Valenstein, E. (eds.) 1979. *Clinical Neuropsychology*. New York: Oxford University Press.

Heilman, K.M. & Watson, R.T. 1977. The neglect syndrome—a unilateral defect of the orienting response. In Harnad, Doty, Goldstein, Jaynes & Krauthamer (1977).

Hermelin, B. & O'Conner, N. 1971. Functional asymmetry in the reading of Braille. *Neuropsychologia, 9*, 431-35.

Herron, J. (ed.) 1980. *Neuropsychology of Left-Handedness*. New York: Academic Press.

Hicks, R.A., Pelligrini, R.J. & Evans, E.A. 1978. Handedness and birth risk. *Neuropsychologia, 16*, 243-45.

Hilgard, J.R. 1979. *Personality and Hypnosis*, second edition. Chicago: University of Chicago Press.

Hines, D. 1977. Differences in tachistoscopic recognition between abstract and concrete words as a function of visual half-field and frequency. *Cortex, 13*, 66-73.

Hiscock, M. & Kinsbourne, M. 1978. Ontogeny of cerebral dominance: evidence from time-sharing asymmetry in children. *Developmental Psychology, 14*, 321-29.

Hiscock, M. & Kinsbourne, M. 1980. Asymmetry of verbal-manual time sharing in children: a followup study. *Neuropsychologia, 18*, 151-62.

Hochberg, F.H. & LeMay, M. 1975. Arteriographic correlates of handedness. *Neurology, 25,* 218-22.

Hoffman, H.J., Hendrick, E.B., Dennis, M. & Armstrong, D. 1979. Hemispherectomy for Sturge-Weber Syndrome. *Child's Brain, 5,* 233-48.

Hoffman, C. & Kagan, S. 1977. Lateral eye movements and field-dependence-independence. *Perceptual and Motor Skills, 45,* 767-78.

Hoppe, K.D. 1977. Split brains and psychoanalysis. *The Psychoanalytic Quarterly, 46,* 220-24.

Humphrey, M.E. & Zangwill, O.L. 1951. Cessation of dreaming after brain injury. *Journal of Neurology, Neurosurgery, and Psychiatry, 14,* 322-25.

Huttenlocher, P.R. 1979. Synaptic density in human frontal cortex— developmental changes and effects of aging. *Brain Research, 163,* 195-205.

Inglis, J. & Lawson, J.S. 1981. Sex differences in the effects of unilateral brain damage on intelligence. *Science, 212,* 693-95.

Ingram, D. 1975. Motor asymmetries in young children. *Neuropsychologia, 13,* 95-102.

Ingvar, D.H. 1976. Functional landscapes of the dominant hemisphere. *Brain Research, 107,* 181-97.

Isaacson, R.L. 1975. The myth of recovery from early brain damage. In N.E. Ellis (ed.) *Aberrant Development in Infancy.* London: Wiley.

Jackendoff, R. mimeo. Generative music theory and its relevance to psychology. Presented at APA, Toronto, 1978. Brandeis University: mimeo.

Jackson, J.H. 1915. On the nature of the duality of the brain. *Brain, 38,* 80-103.

Jacobson, M.J. 1978. *Developmental Neurobiology,* second edition. New York: Plenum Press.

Jaynes, J. 1976. *The Origins of Consciousness in the Breakdown of the Bicameral Mind.* Boston: Houghton Mifflin.

Jensen, A.R. 1975. A theoretical note on sex linkage and race differences in spatial visualization ability. *Behavior Genetics, 5,* 151-64.

John, E.R. 1971. Brain mechanisms of memory. In J.L. McGaugh (ed.) *Psychobiology.* New York: Academic Press.

Johnson, D.D. 1973. Sex differences in reading across cultures. *Reading Research Quarterly, 9* (1), 67–86.

Johnson, O. & Kozma, A. 1977. Effects of concurrent verbal and musical tasks on a unimanual skill. *Cortex, 13,* 11–16.

Jones, R.K. 1966. Observations on stammering after localized cerebral injury. *Journal of Neurology, Neurosurgery, and Psychiatry, 29,* 192–95.

Katz, A.N. 1979. Creativity and the cerebral hemispheres. *American Psychologist, 34,* 279–80.

Kershner, J.R. 1977. Good readers and gifted children: search for a valid model. *Child Development, 48,* 61–67.

Kertesz, A. 1979. *Aphasia and Associated Disorders: Taxonomy: Localization, and Recovery.* New York: Grune & Stratton.

Kertesz, A., Lesk, D. & McCabe, P. 1977. Isotope localization of infarcts in aphasia. *Archives of Neurology, 34,* 590–601.

Kimura, D. 1961a. Some effects of temporal-lobe damage on auditory perception. *Canadian Journal of Psychology, 15,* 156–65.

Kimura, D. 1961b. Cerebral dominance and the perception of verbal stimuli. *Canadian Journal of Psychology, 15,* 166–75.

Kimura, D. 1967. Functional asymmetry of the brain in dichotic listening. *Cortex, 3,* 163–78.

Kimura, D. 1969. Spatial localization in left and right visual fields. *Canadian Journal of Psychology, 23,* 445–58.

Kimura, D. 1973. Manual activity during speaking—I. Right-handers. *Neuropsychologia, 11,* 45–50.

Kimura, D. 1974. Left-right differences in the perception of melodies. *Quarterly Journal of Experimental Psychology, 16,* 355–58.

Kimura, D. 1976. The neural basis of language qua gesture. In H. Whitaker & H.A. Whitaker (eds.) *Studies in Neurolinguistics: Volume 2.* New York: Academic Press.

Kimura, D. 1977. Acquisition of a motor skill after left-hemisphere damage. *Brain, 100,* 527–42.

Kimura, D. & Archibald, Y. 1974. Motor functions of the left hemisphere. *Brain, 97,* 337–50.

Kimura, D. & Folb, S. 1968. Neural processing of backwards speech sounds. *Science, 161,* 395–96.

King, F.L. & Kimura, D. 1972. Left-ear superiority in dichotic perception of vocal nonverbal sounds. *Canadian Journal of Psychology, 26,* 111–16.

Kinsbourne, M. 1971. The minor hemisphere as a source of aphasic speech. *Archives of Neurology, 25*, 302–06.
Kinsbourne, M. 1972. Eye and head turning indicates cerebral lateralization. *Science, 176*, 539–41.
Kinsbourne, M. 1974. Direction of gaze and distribution of cerebral thought processes. *Neuropsychologia, 12*, 279–81.
Kinsbourne, M. 1978. Evolution of language in relation to lateral action. In M. Kinsbourne (ed.) *Asymmetrical Function of the Brain.* Cambridge: Cambridge University Press.
Kinsbourne, M. 1979. Language lateralization and developmental disorders. In C.L. Ludlow & M.E. Doran-Quine (eds.) *The Neurological Bases of Language Disorders in Children: Methods and Directions for Research.* Bethesda: NINCDS Monograph Series.
Kinsbourne, M. & Cook, J. 1971. Generalized and lateralized effects of concurrent verbalization on a unimanual skill. *Quarterly Journal of Experimental Psychology, 23*, 341–45.
Kinsbourne, M. & Hicks, E. 1978. Functional cerebral space: a model for overflow, transfer and interference effects in human performance: a tutorial review. In J. Requin (ed.) *Attention and Performance VII.* Hillsdale, NJ: Lawrence Erlbaum.
Kinsbourne, M. & Hiscock, M. 1977. Does cerebral dominance develop? In Segalowitz & Gruber (1977a).
Kinsbourne, M. & Lempert, H. 1979. Does left brain lateralization of speech arise from right-biased orienting to salient percepts? *Human Development: 22*, 270–76.
Kitchener, R.F. 1978. Epigenesis: the role of biological models in developmental psychology. *Human Development, 21*, 141–60.
Kitchener, R.F. 1980. Predetermined versus probabilistic epigenesis. *Human Development, 23*, 73–76.
Kohn, B. & Dennis, M. 1974a. Selective impairments of visuo-spatial abilities in infantile hemiplegia after right cerebral hemidecortication. *Neuropsychologia, 12*, 505–12.
Kohn, B. & Dennis, M. 1974b. Patterns of hemispheric specialization after hemidecortication for infantile hemiplegia. In M. Kinsbourne & L. Smith (eds.) *Hemispheric Disconnection and Cerebral Function.* Springfield, IL: Charles C. Thomas.
Kolb, B. & Whishaw, I.Q. 1980. *Fundamentals of Human Neuropsychology.* San Francisco: W.H. Freeman.

Kotik, B.S. 1979. An investigation of speech lateralization in multi-linguals. (In Russian) *Voprosii Psikhologii*, 74–78.

Krashen, S.D. 1973. Lateralization, language learning, and the critical period: some new evidence. *Language Learning, 23*, 63–74.

Krashen, S.D. 1976. Cerebral asymmetry. In H. Whitaker & H.A. Whitaker (eds.) *Studies in Neurolinguistics, vol. 2*. New York: Academic Press.

Krech, D. 1962. Cortical localization of function. In L. Postman (ed.) *Psychology in the Making*. New York: Alfred A. Knopf.

Kuhl, P.K. & Miller, J.D. 1975. Speech perception by the chinchilla: the voiced-voiceless distinction in alveolar plosive consonants. *Science, 190*, 69–72.

Lackner, J. & Teuber, H. 1973. Alterations in auditory fusion thresholds after cerebral injury in man. *Neuropsychologia, 11*, 409–15.

Lake, D. & Bryden, M.P. 1976. Handedness and sex differences in hemispheric asymmetry. *Brain and Language, 3*, 266–82.

Lansdell, H. 1964. Sex differences in hemispheric asymmetries of the human brain. *Nature, 203*, 550.

Lansdell, H. 1973. Effect of neurosurgery on the ability to identify popular word associations. *Journal of Abnormal Psychology, 81*, 255–58.

Lassen, N.A., Ingvar, D.H. & Skinhoj, E. 1978. Brain function and blood flow. *Scientific American*, October 1978, 62–71.

Lawson, N.C. 1978. Inverted writing in right- and left-handers in relation to lateralization of face recognition. *Cortex, 14*, 207–11.

LeMay, M. & Culebras, A. 1972. Human brain-morphologic differences in the hemispheres demonstrable by carotid arteriography. *New England Journal of Medicine, 287*, 168–70.

LeMay, M. & Geschwind, N. 1975. Hemispheric differences in the brains of great apes. *Brain, Behavior and Evolution, 11*, 48–52.

Lenneberg, E.H. 1967. *Biological Foundation of Language*. New York: Wiley.

Lenneberg, E.H. 1975. In search of a dynamic theory of aphasia. In E.H. Lenneberg & E. Lenneberg (eds.) *Foundations of Language Development, Vol. 2*. New York: Academic Press.

Lerner, R.M. 1976. *Concepts and Theories of Human Development*. Reading, MA: Addison-Wesley.

Lerner, R.M. 1980. Concepts of epigenesis: descriptive and explanatory issues. *Human Development, 23,* 63-72.

Levy, J. 1969. Possible basis for the evolution of lateral specialization of the human brain. *Nature, 224,* 614-15.

Levy, J. 1977. The mammalian brain and the adaptive advantage of cerebral asymmetry. *Annals of the New York Academy of Sciences, 299,* 264-72.

Levy, J. & Nagylaki, T. 1972. A model for the genetics of handedness. *Genetics, 72,* 117-28.

Levy, J. & Reid, M. 1976. Variations in writing posture and cerebral organization. *Science, 194,* 337-39.

Levy, J. & Reid, M. 1978. Variations in cerebral organization as a function of handedness, hand posture in writing, and sex. *Journal of Experimental Psychology: General, 107,* 119-44.

Ley, R. 1980a. Emotion and the right hemisphere. Unpublished dissertation, University of Waterloo.

Ley, R. 1980b. An archival examination of an asymmetry of hysterical conversion symptoms. *Journal of Clinical Neuropsychology, 2,* 1-9.

Ley, R.G. & Bryden, M.P. 1979. Hemispheric differences in recognizing faces and emotions. *Brain and Language, 7,* 127-38.

Ley, R.G. & Bryden, M.P. 1981. Consciousness, emotion, and the right hemisphere. In G. Underwood & S. Stevens (eds.) *Aspects of Consciousness.* New York: Academic Press.

Liberman, A., Cooper, F., Shankweiler, D. & Studdert-Kennedy, M. 1967. Perception and the speech code. *Psychological Review, 74,* 431-61.

Lieberman, P. 1975. *On the Origins of Language: An Introduction to the Evolution of Human Speech.* New York: Macmillan.

Linden, E. 1974. *Apes and Men.* New York: Penguin.

Lishman, W.A. & McMeekan, E. 1977. Handedness in relation to direction and degree of cerebral fominance for language. *Cortex, 13,* 30-43.

Lisker, L. & Abramson, A.S. 1964. A cross-language study of voicing in initial stops: acoustical measurements. *Word, 20,* 384-422.

Lomas, J. & Kimura, D. 1976. Interhemispheric interaction between speaking and sequential manual activity. *Neuropsychologia, 14,* 23-33.

Luria, A.R. 1963. *Restoration of Function After Brain Injury.* New York: Macmillan.

Luria, A.R. 1966a. *Higher Cortical Functions.* New York: Basic Books.

Luria, A.R. 1966b. *Human Brain and Psychological Processes.* New York: Harper & Row.

Luria, A.R. 1969. On the pathology of computational operations. In J. Kilpatrick & I. Wirszup (eds.) *Soviet Studies in the Psychology of Learning and Teaching Mathematics: Vol. 1 The Learning of Mathematics.* Chicago: University of Chicago Press.

Luria, A.R. 1970a. The functional organization of the brain. *Scientific American, 222,* 6-78.

Luria, A.R. 1970b. *Traumatic Aphasia.* The Hague: Mouton.

Luria, A.R., Tsvetkova, L.S. & Futer, D. 1965. Aphasia in a composer. *Journal of the Neurological Sciences, 2,* 288-92.

Maccoby, E.E. & Jacklin, C.N. 1974. *The Psychology of Sex Differences.* Stanford: Stanford University Press.

Malgady, R.G. 1977. Children's interpretation and appreciation of similes. *Child Development, 48,* 1734-38.

Marcel, T., Katz, L. & Smith, M. 1974. Laterality and reading proficiency. *Neuropsychologia, 12,* 131-39.

Marcel, T. & Rajan, P. 1975. Lateral specialization of words and faces in good and poor readers. *Neuropsychologia, 13,* 489-97.

Marshall, J. 1973. Some problems and paradoxes associated with recent accounts of hemispheric specialization. *Neuropsychologia, 11,* 463-70.

Mason, J.W. 1972. Organization of psychoendocrine mechanisms; a review and reconsideration of research. In N.S. Greenfield & R.A. Sternbach (eds.) *Handbook of Psychophysiology.* New York: Holt, Rinehart, and Winston.

Mavlov, L. 1980. Amusia due to rhythm agnosia in a musician with left hemisphere damage: a non-auditory suprasegmental defect. *Cortex, 16,* 331-38.

McFarland, K. & Ashton, R. 1978. The influence of brain lateralization of function on a manual skill. *Cortex, 14,* 102-11.

McFarland, K., McFarland, M.L., Bain, J.D. & Ashton, R. 1978. Ear differences of abstract and concrete word recognition. *Neuropsychologia, 16,* 555-61.

McGee, M.G. 1979. Human spatial abilities: psychometric studies and environmental, genetic, hormonal, and neurological influences. *Psychological Bulletin, 86,* 889–918.

McGhee, P.E. 1974. Cognitive mastery and children's humor. *Psychological Bulletin, 81,* 721–30.

McGlone, J. 1977. Sex differences in the cerebral organization of verbal functions in patients with unilateral brain lesions. *Brain,* 100, 775–93.

McGlone, J. 1978. Sex differences in functional brain asymmetry. *Cortex, 14,* 122–28.

McGlone, J. 1980. Sex differences in human brain asymmetry: a critical survey. *The Behavioral and Brain Sciences, 3,* 215–63.

McGlone, J. & Kertesz, A. 1973. Sex differences in cerebral processing of visuospatial tasks. *Cortex, 9,* 313–20.

McKeever, W.F. 1981. Evidence against the hypothesis of right hemisphere language dominance in the native American Navajo. *Neuropsychologia, 19,* 595–98.

McKeever, W.F., Hoemann, H.W., Florian, V.A. & Van Deventer, A.D. 1976. Evidence of minimal cerebral asymmetries for the processing of English words and American Sign Language in the congenitally deaf. *Neuropsychologia, 14,* 413–23.

McKeever, W.F. & Huling, M.D. 1971. Lateral dominance in tachistoscopic word recognition performances obtained with simultaneous bilateral input. *Neuropsychologia, 9,* 15–20.

McKeever, W.F. & VanDeventer, A.D. 1975. Dyslexic adolescents: evidence of impaired visual and auditory language processing associated with normal lateralization and visual responsivity. *Cortex, 11,* 361–78.

McKeever, W.F. & VanDeventer, A.D. 1980. Inverted handwriting position, language laterality and the Levy-Nagylaki genetic model of handedness and cerebral organization. *Neuropsychologia, 18,* 99–102.

Mebert, C.J. & Michel, G.F. 1980. Handedness in artists. In Herron (1980).

Miceli, G., Caltagirone, C., Gainotti, G. & Payer-Rigo, P. 1978. Discrimination of voice versus place contrasts in aphasia. *Brain and Language, 6,* 47–51.

Mills, L. & Rollman, G.B. 1979. Left hemisphere selectivity for processing duration in normal subjects. *Brain and Language,* 7, 320-35.

Milner, B. 1962. Laterality effects in audition. In V. Mountcastle (ed.) *Interhemispheric Relations and Cerebral Dominance.* Baltimore: Johns Hopkins University Press.

Milner, B. 1967. Comments on Rossi & Rosadini, p. 177. In C.H. Millikan & F.L. Darley (eds.) *Brain Mechanisms Underlying Speech and Language.* New York: Grune & Stratton.

Mitchell, D. & Blakemore, C. 1969. Binocular depth perception and the corpus callosum. *Vision Research, 10,* 49-54.

Molfese, D.L. 1978a. Left and right hemisphere involvement in speech perception: electrophysiological correlates. *Perception & Psychophysics, 23,* 237-43.

Molfese, D.L. 1978b. Neuroelectrical correlates of categorical perception in adults. *Brain and Language, 5,* 25-35.

Molfese, D.L. 1979. Cortical involvement in the semantic processing of coarticulated speech cues. *Brain and Language, 7,* 86-100.

Molfese, D.L. 1980a. The phoneme and the engram: electrophysiological evidence for the acoustic invariant in stop consonants. *Brain and Language, 9,* 372-76.

Molfese, D.L. 1980b. Hemispheric specialization for temporal information: implications for the perception of voicing cues during speech perception. *Brain and Language, 11,* 285-99.

Molfese, D.L., Freeman, R.B. & Palermo, D.S. 1975. The ontogeny of brain lateralization for speech and nonspeech stimuli. *Brain and Language, 2,* 356-68.

Molfese, D.L. & Molfese, V.J. 1979a. Hemisphere and stimulus differences as reflected in the cortical responses of newborn infants to speech stimuli. *Developmental Psychology, 15,* 505-11.

Molfese, D.L. & Molfese, V.J. 1979b. VOT distinctions in infants: learned or innate? In H. Whitaker & H.A. Whitaker (eds.) *Studies in Neurolinguistics Vol. 4.* New York: Academic Press.

Moore, W.H., Jr., & Haynes, W.O. 1980. A study of alpha hemispheric asymmetries for verbal and nonverbal stimuli in males and females. *Brain and Language, 9,* 338-49.

Morgan, M.J. & Corballis, M.C. 1978. On the biological basis of human laterality: II. The mechanisms of inheritance. *The Behavioral and Brain Sciences, 2,* 270-77.

Morgan, A.H., McDonald, F.J. & MacDonald, H. 1971. Differences in bilateral alpha activity as a function of experimental task, with a note on lateral eye-movements and hypnotizability. *Neuropsychologia, 9,* 459-69.

Moscovitch, M. 1977. The development of lateralization of language and its relation to cognitive and linguistic development: a review and some theoretical speculations. In Segalowitz & Gruber (1977a).

Moscovitch, M. & Olds, J. 1982. Asymmetries in spontaneous facial expressions and their possible relation to hemispheric specialization. *Neuropsychologia, 20,* 71-81.

Moscovitch, M. & Smith, L.C. 1979. Differences in neural organization between individuals with inverted and noninverted handwriting postures. *Science, 205,* 710-13.

Mosidze, V.M. 1976. On the lateralization of musical function in man. [in Russian] In V.P. Kaznacheyev, S.F. Semyonov & A.P. Chuprikov (eds.) *Functional Asymmetry and Adaptation in Man.* Moscow.

Moss, H. 1967. Sex, age and state as determinants of mother-infant interactions. *The Merrill-Palmer Quarterly, 13,* 19-36.

Moss, H. 1973. Talk presented at Cornell University, Department of Human Development and Family Studies.

Myers, R.E. 1962. Transmission of visual information within and between the hemispheres: a behavioral study. In V.B. Mountcastle (ed.) *Interhemispheric Relations and Cerebral Dominance.* Baltimore: Johns Hopkins University Press.

Myslobodsky, M.S. & Rattok, J. 1977. Bilateral electrodermal activity in waking man. *Acta Psychologica, 41,* 273-82.

Nachshon, I. 1973. Effects of cerebral dominance and attention on dichotic listening. *T-I-T Journal of Life Sciences, 3,* 107-14.

Nachshon, I. 1978. Handedness and dichotic listening to nonverbal features of speech. *Perceptual and Motor Skills, 47,* 1111-14.

Nash, J. 1970. *Developmental Psychology: a Psychobiological Approach.* Englewood Cliffs: Prentice-Hall.

Naylor, H. 1980. Reading disability and lateral asymmetry: an information-processing analysis. *Psychological Bulletin, 87,* 531-45.

Nebes, R.D. 1974. Hemispheric specialization in commissuroto-mized man. *Psychological Bulletin, 81,* 1-14.

Neisser, U. 1976. *Cognition and Reality.* San Francisco: W.H. Freeman.

Netley, C. 1977. Dichotic listening of callosal agenesis and Turner's syndrome patients. In Segalowitz & Gruber (1977a).

Newcombe, F. & Ratcliffe, G. 1973. Handedness, speech lateraliza-tion and ability. *Neuropsychologia, 11,* 399-407.

Nottebohm, F. 1977. Asymmetries in neural control of vocalization in the canary. In Harnad, Doty, Goldstein, Jaynes & Kraut-hamer (1977).

Nottebohm, F. 1979. Origins and mechanisms in the establishment of cerebral dominance. In M.S. Gazzaniga (ed.) *Handbook of Behavioral Neurobiology, Vol. 2.* New York: Plenum.

Nottebohm, F. 1980. Testosterone triggers growth of brain vocal control nuclei in adult female canaries. *Brain Research, 189,* 429-36.

Nottebohm, F. & Arnold, A.P. 1976. Sexual dimorphism in vocal control areas of the songbird brain. *Science, 194,* 211-13.

O'Brien, B. 1958. *Operators and Things: The Inner Life of a Schizo-phrenic.* London: Elek.

Ojemann, G.A. & Whitaker, H.A. 1978. Language localization and variability. *Brain and Language, 6,* 239-60.

Oldfield, R.C. 1969. Handedness in musicians.

Oldfield, R.C. 1971. The assessment and analysis of handedness: The Edinburgh Inventory. *Neuropsychologia, 9,* 97-113.

Oltman, P.K. 1979. Cognitive style and interhemispheric differentia-tion in the EEG. *Neuropsychologia, 17,* 699-702.

Oltman, P.K., Ehrlichman, H. & Cox, P.W. 1977. Field independence and laterality in the perception of faces. *Perceptual and Motor Skills, 45,* 255-60.

Ornstein, R. 1972. *The Psychology of Consciousness.* New York: The Viking Press.

Ornstein, R. & Galin, D. 1976. Physiological studies of conscious-ness. In P.R. Lee, R. Ornstein, D. Galin, A. Deikman & C. Tart (eds.) *Symposium on Consciousness.* New York: Viking Press.

Orr, C. 1980. Exploring the relationships between psychological differentiation and cerebral lateralization. Unpublished Honours Thesis, Brock University.

Orton, S.T. 1937. *Reading, Writing and Speech Problems in Children.* New York: W.W. Norton.

Paivio, A. 1971. *Imagery and Verbal Processes.* New York: Holt, Rinehart & Winston.

Paradis, M. 1977. Bilingualism and aphasia. In H. Whitaker & H.A. Whitaker (eds.) *Studies in Neurolinguistics, Vol. 3.* New York: Academic Press.

Paradis, M. 1980. Alternate antagonism with paradoxical translation behavior in two bilingual aphasic patients. Paper presented at BABBLE, Niagara Falls, Ontario.

Paredes, J.A. & Hepburn, M.J. 1976. The split brain and the culture-and-cognition paradox. *Current Anthropology, 17,* 121–27.

Park, S. & Arbuckle, T.Y. 1977. Ideograms versus alphabets: effects of script on memory in "biscriptual" Korean subjects. *Journal of Experimental Psychology: Human Learning and Memory, 3,* 631–42.

Parsons, J. (ed.) 1980. *The Psychobiology of Sex Differences and Sex Roles.* Washington, D.C.: Hemisphere Publishing.

Pavlidis, G. Th. 1981. Do eye movements hold the key to dyslexia? *Neuropsychologia, 19,* 57–64.

Penfield, W. & Roberts, L. 1959. *Speech and Brain Mechanisms.* Princeton, NJ: Princeton University Press.

Peters, M. & Petrie, B. 1979. Functional asymmetry in the stepping reflex of human neonates. *Canadian Journal of Psychology, 33,* 198–200.

Peterson, A.C. 1976. Physical androgyny and cognitive functioning in adolescence. *Developmental Psychology, 12,* 524–33.

Peterson, A.C. 1979. Hormones and cognitive functioning in normal development. In Wittig & Peterson (1979).

Peterson, J.M. & Lansky, L.M. 1974. Left-handedness among architects: some facts and speculation. *Perceptual and Motor Skills, 38,* 547–50.

Peterson, J.M. & Lansky, L.M. 1977. Left-handedness among architects: partial replication and some new data. *Perceptual and Motor Skills, 45,* 1216–18.

Petrie, B. & Peters, M. 1979. Motor asymmetries in infants. Presented at the Canadian Psychological Association, Quebec, Quebec.

Pettito, L.A. & Seidenberg, M.S. 1979. On the evidence for linguistic abilities in signing apes. *Brain and Language, 8,* 162–83.

Piazza, D.M. 1977. Cerebral lateralization in young children as measured by dichotic listening and finger tapping tasks. *Neuropsychologia, 15,* 417-25.

Piazza, D.M. 1980. The influence of sex and handedness in the hemispheric specialization of verbal and nonverbal tasks. *Neuropsychologia, 18,* 163-76.

Pizzamiglio, L. 1974. Handedness, ear-preference and field dependence. *Perceptual and Motor Skills, 38,* 700-02.

Poizner, H., Battison, R. & Lane, H. 1979. Cerebral asymmetry for American Sign Language: the effects of moving stimuli. *Brain and Language, 7,* 351-62.

Porac, C., Coren, S. & Duncan, P. 1980. Life-span age trends in laterality. *Journal of Gerontology, 35,* 715-21.

Poizner, H. & Lane, H. 1979. Cerebral asymmetry in the perception of American Sign Language. *Brain and Language, 7,* 210-26.

Porter, R.J. & Berlin, C.I. 1975. On interpreting developmental changes in the dichotic right-ear advantage. *Brain and Language, 2,* 186-200.

Prohovnik, I., Hakansson, K. & Risberg, J. 1980. Observations on the functional significance of regional cerebral blood flow in "resting" normal subjects. *Neuropsychologia, 18,* 203-17.

Provins, K.A. & Glencross, D.J. 1968. Handwriting, typewriting and handedness. *Quarterly Journal of Experimental Psychology, 20,* 282-89.

Rasmussen, T. & Milner, B. 1977. The role of early left-brain injury in determining lateralization of cerebral speech functions. *Annals of the New York Academy of Sciences, 299,* 355-69.

Ray, W.J., Morell, M., Frediani, A.W. & Tucker, D. 1976. Sex differences and lateral specialization of hemispheric functioning. *Neuropsychologia, 14,* 391-94.

Rimland, B. 1964. *Infantile Autism: the Syndrome and its Implications for a Neural Theory of Behavior.* Englewood Cliffs: Prentice-Hall.

Rimland, B. 1978. Inside the mind of the autistic savant. *Psychology Today, 12,* 69-80.

Risberg, J. & Ingvar, D.H. 1973. Patterns of activation in the grey matter of the dominant hemisphere during memorizing and reasoning, *Brain, 96,* 737-56.

Risse, G., LeDoux, J., Springer, S.P., Wilson, D.H. & Gazzaniga, M. 1978. The anterior commissure in man: functional variation in a multisensory system. *Neuropsychologia, 16,* 23-31.

Rizzolatti, G., Bertoloni, G. & Buchtel, H.A. 1979. Interface of concomitant motor and verbal tasks on simple reaction time: a hemispheric difference. *Neuropsychologia, 17,* 323-30.

Robinson, G.M. & Solomon, D.J. 1974. Rhythm is processed by the speech hemisphere. *Journal of Experimental Psychology, 102,* 508-11.

Robinson, R.G. 1979. Differential behavioral and biochemical effects of right and left hemispheric cerebral infarction in the rat. *Science, 205,* 707-10.

Roemer, R.A., Shagass, C., Strumanis, J.J. & Amadeo, M. 1978. Pattern evoked potential measurements suggesting lateralized hemispheric dysfunction in chronic schizophrenics. *Biological Psychiatry, 13,* 185-202.

Rogers, L., TenHouten, W., Kaplan, C.D. & Gardiner, M. 1977. Hemispheric specialization of language: an EEG study of bilingual Hopi Indian children. *International Journal of Neuroscience, 8,* 1-6.

Rose, S. 1976. *The Conscious Brain,* updated edition. New York: Random House.

Rose, S. & Rose, H. 1973. 'Do not adjust your mind, there is a fault in reality'—ideology in neurobiology, *Cognition, 2,* 479-502.

Rosenzweig, M.R. 1951. Representation of the two ears at the auditory cortex. *American Journal of Physiology, 167,* 147-58.

Rosenzweig, M.R. 1979. Responsiveness of brain size to individual experience: behavioral and evolutionary implications. In M.E. Hahn, C. Jensen & B.C. Dudek (eds.) *Development and Evolution of Brain Size: Behavioral Implications.* New York: Academic Press.

Rosenthal, R. & Bigelow, L.B. 1972. Quantitative brain measurements in chronic schizophrenia. *British Journal of Psychiatry, 121,* 259-64.

Ross, E.D. & Mesulam, M.M. 1979. Dominant language functions of the right hemisphere? *Archives of Neurology, 36,* 144-48.

Ross, P. (in press). Cerebral asymmetries in deaf individuals. In Segalowitz (1983).

Ross, P., Pergament, L. & Anisfeld, M. 1979. Cerebral lateralization of deaf and hearing individuals for linguistic comparison judgments. *Brain and Language, 8,* 69–80.

Ross, P. & Turkewitz, G. in press. Individual differences in cerebral asymmetries for facial recognition. *Cortex.*

Rossi, G.F. & Rosadini, G. 1967. Experimental analysis of cerebral dominance in man. In C.H. Millikan & F.L. Darley (eds.) *Brain Mechanisms Underlying Speech and Language.* New York: Grune & Stratton.

Rourke, B.P. 1978. Neuropsychological research in reading retardation: a review. In A.L. Benton & D. Pearl (eds.) *Dyslexia: An Appraisal of Current Knowledge.* New York: Oxford University Press.

Rozin, P., Poritsky, S. & Sotsky, R. 1971. American children with reading problems can easily learn to read English represented by Chinese characters. *Science, 171,* 1264–67.

Rubens, A.B. 1977. Anatomical asymmetries of human cerebral cortex. In Harnad, Doty, Goldstein, Jaynes & Krauthamer (1977).

Rubens, A.B. 1979. Agnosia. In Heilman & Valenstein (1979).

Rudel, R.G., Denckla, M.B. & Spalten, E. 1974. The functional asymmetry of Braille letter learning in normal, sighted children. *Neurology, 24,* 733–38.

Russell, B. 1946. *History of Western Philosophy.* London: Allen & Unwin.

St. James-Roberts, I. 1979. Neurological plasticity, recovery from brain insult, and child development. *Advances in Child Development and Behavior, 14,* 253–319.

St. James-Roberts, I. 1981. A reinterpretation of hemispherectomy data without functional plasticity of the brain. *Brain and Language, 13,* 31–53.

Sameroff, A.J. 1975. Early influences on development: fact or fancy? *Merrill-Palmer Quarterly, 21,* 267–94.

Samuels, J.A. & Benson, D.F. 1979. Some aspects of language comprehension in anterior aphasics. *Brain and Language, 8,* 275–86.

Sasanuma, S. 1975. Kana and Kanji processing in Japanese aphasics. *Brain and Language, 2,* 369–83.

Sasanuma, S., Itoh, M., Mori, K. & Kobayashi, Y. 1977. Tachisto-scopic recognition of Kana and Kanji words. *Neuropsychologia, 15,* 547–53.

Satz, P. 1972. Pathological left-handedness: an explanatory model. *Cortex, 8,* 121–35.

Satz, P. 1977. Laterality tests: an inferential problem. *Cortex, 13,* 208–12.

Satz, P., Fennel, E. & Jones, M.B. 1969. Comments on: A model of inheritance of handedness and cerebral dominance. *Neuropsychologia, 7,* 101–03.

Schaller, G.B. 1963. *The Mountain Gorilla.* Chicago: The University of Chicago Press.

Schneider, G.E. 1979. Is it really better to have your brain lesion early? A revision of the "Kennard principle." *Neuropsychologia, 17,* 557–83.

Scholes, R.J. & Fischler, I. 1979. Hemispheric function and linguistic skill in the deaf. *Brain and Language, 7,* 336–50.

Schucard, D.W., Schucard, J.L. & Thomas, D.G. 1977. Auditory evoked potentials as probes of hemispheric diffe ences in cognitive processing. *Science, 197,* 1295–98.

Schwartz, G.E., Davidson, R.J. & Maer, F. 1975. Right hemispheric lateralization for emotion in the human brain: interactions with cognition. *Science, 190,* 286–88.

Schwartz, J. & Tallal, P. 1980. Rate of acoustic change may underlie hemispheric specialization for speech perception. *Science, 207,* 1380–81.

Schwartz, M. 1977. Left-handedness and high-risk pregnancy. *Neuropsychologia, 15,* 341–44.

Scott, S., Hynd, G.W., Hunt, L. & Weed, W. 1979. Cerebral speech lateralization in the native American Navajo. *Neuropsychologia, 17,* 89–92.

Searle, J. 1969. *Speech Acts.* Cambridge: Cambridge University Press.

Segalowitz, N.S. & Hansson, P. 1979. Hemispheric fun processing of agent-patient information. *Brain* 8, 51–61.

Segalowitz, S.J. 1980. Review of *The Integr Language, 11,* 225–28.

Segalowitz, S.J. mimeo. Developmental models of brain lateralization. Mimeo, Brock University, St. Catharines, Ontario.

Segalowitz, S.J. (ed.) 1983. *Language Functions and Brain Organization*. New York: Academic Press.

Segalowitz, S.J., Bebout, L.J. & Lederman, S.J. 1979. Lateralization for reading musical chords: disentangling symbolic, analytic, and phonological aspects of reading. *Brain and Language, 8*, 315–23.

Segalowitz, S.J., & Bryden, M.P. in press. Individual differences in hemispheric representation of language. In Segalowitz (in press).

Segalowitz, S.J. & Chapman, J.S. 1980. Cerebral asymmetry for speech in neonates: a behavioral measure. *Brain and Language, 9*, 281–88.

Segalowitz, S.J. & Gruber, F.A. (eds.) 1977a. *Language Development and Neurological Theory*. New York: Academic Press.

Segalowitz, S.J. & Gruber, F.A. 1977b. What is it that is lateralized? In Segalowitz & Gruber (1977a).

Segalowitz, S.J. & Gruber, F.A. 1977c. Why is language lateralized to the left? In Segalowitz & Gruber (1977a).

Segalowitz, S.J. & Orr, C. 1981. How to measure individual differences in brain lateralization: demonstration of a paradigm. Presented at INS, Atlanta, GA.

Segalowitz, S.J. & Stewart, C. 1979. Left and right lateralization for letter matching: strategy and sex differences. *Neuropsychologia, 17*, 521–25.

Selfe, L. 1977. *Nadia: a case of extraordinary drawing ability in an autistic child*. New York: Academic Press.

Semmes, J. 1968. Hemispheric specialization: a possible clue to mechanism. *Neuropsychologia, 6*, 11–26.

Seth, G. 1973. Eye-hand co-ordination and "handedness": a developmental study of visuo-motor behaviour in infancy. *British Journal of Educational Psychology, 43*, 35–49.

Shankweiler, D. & Studdert-Kennedy, M. 1967. Identification of consonants and vowels presented to left and right ears. *Quarterly Journal of Experimental Psychology, 19*, 59–63.

Shankweiler, D. & Studdert-Kennedy, M. 1975. A continuum of lateralization for speech perception? *Brain and Language, 2*, 25.

Shanon, B. 1978. Writing position in Americans and Israelis. *Neuropsychologia, 16*, 587-91.

Shultz, T.R. 1974. Development of the appreciation of riddles. *Child Development, 45*, 100-05.

Sidtis, J.J. 1980. On the nature of the cortical function underlying right hemisphere auditory perception. *Neuropsychologia, 18*, 321-30.

Smith, A. 1966. Speech and other functions after left (dominant) hemispherectomy. *Journal of Neurology, Neurosurgery and Psychiatry, 29*, 467-71.

Smith, C. & Lloyd, B. 1978. Maternal behavior and perceived sex of infant: revisited. *Child Development, 49*, 1263-65.

Smith, M.O., Chu, J. & Edmonston, W.E. 1977. Cerebral lateralization of haptic perception: interaction of responses to Braille and music reveals a functional basis. *Science, 197*, 689-90.

Sparks, R. & Geschwind, N. 1968. Dichotic listening in man after section of neocortical commissures.*Cortex, 4*, 3-16.

Sparks, R., Helm, N. & Albert, M. 1974. Aphasia rehabilitation resulting from melodic intonation therapy. *Cortex, 10*, 303-16.

Spellacy, F. & Blumstein, S. 1970. The influence of language set on ear preference in phoneme recognition. *Cortex, 6*, 430-39.

Sperry, R.W. 1968. Hemisphere deconnection and unity in conscious awareness. *American Psychologist, 23*, 723-33.

Spreen, O., Benton, A.L. & Fincham, R.W. 1965. Auditory agnosia without aphasia. *Archives of Neurology, 13*, 84-92.

Stein, D.G., Rosen, J.J. & Butters, N. (eds.) 1974. *Plasticity and recovery of function in the central nervous system.* New York: Academic Press.

Studdert-Kennedy, M. & Shankweiler, D. 1970. Hemispheric specialization for speech perception. *Journal of the Acoustical Society of America, 48*, 579-94.

Taub, J.M., Tanguay, P.E., Doubleday, C.N., Clarkson, D. & Remington, R. 1976. Hemisphere and ear asymmetry in the auditory evoked response to musical chord stimuli. *Physiological Psychology, 4*, 11-17.

Taylor, J. 1932. *Selected Writings of John Hughlings Jackson,* 2 vol. London: Hodder & Stroughton.

Terrace, H. 1979. *NIM: a chimpanzee who learned sign language.* New York: Knopf.

Terzian, H. 1964. Behavioral and EEG effects of intracarotid sodium amytal injections. *Acta Neurochirugia, 12,* 230–40.

Trehub, S. 1979. Reflections on the development of speech perception. *Canadian Journal of Psychology. 33,* 368–81.

Tucker, D.M. 1981. Lateral brain function, emotion, and conceptualization. *Psychological Bulletin, 89,* 19–46.

Tucker, D.M., Stenslie, C.E., Roth, R.S. & Shearer, S.L. 1981. Right frontal lobe activation and right hemisphere performance. *Archives of General Psychiatry, 38,* 169–74.

Tucker, D.M., Watson, R.G. & Heilman, K.M. 1976. Affective discrimination and evocation in patients with right parietal disease. *Neurology, 26,* 354.

Tzavara, A., Kaprinis, G. & Gatzoyas, A. 1981. Literacy and hemispheric specialization for language: digit dichotic listening in illiterates. *Neuropsychologia, 19,* 565–70.

Umilta, C., Rizzolatti, G., Marzi, C., Franzini, C., Carmada, R. & Berlucchi, G. 1974. Hemispheric differences in the discrimination of line orientation. *Neuropsychologia, 12,* 165–74.

Uttal, W.R. 1978. *The Psychobiology of Mind.* Hillsdale, NJ: Lawrence Erlbaum Associates.

Vaid, J. & Genesee, F. 1980. Neuropsychological approaches to bilingualism: a critical review. *Canadian Journal of Psychology, 34,* 24–31.

VanLancker, D. 1972. Language lateralization and grammars. *UCLA Working Papers in Phonetics, 23,* 24–31.

VanLancker, D. & Fromkin, V.A. 1973. Hemispheric specialization for pitch and "tone": evidence from Thai. *Journal of Phonetics, 1,* 101–09.

Vargha-Khadem, F. & Corballis, M.C. 1979. Cerebral asymmetry in infants. *Brain and Language, 8,* 1–9.

Waber, D. 1976. Sex differences in cognition: a function of maturation rate? *Science, 192,* 572–74.

Waber, D. 1977. Sex differences in mental abilities, hemispheric lateralization, and rate of physical growth at adolescence. *Developmental Psychology, 13,* 29–38.

Waber, D. 1979. Cognitive abilities and sex-related variations in the maturation of cerebral cortical functions. In Wittig & Peterson (1979).

Wachtel, P.I. 1972. Field dependence and psychological differentiation: a reexamination. *Perceptual and Motor Skills, 35,* 179-89.

Wada, J., Clarke, R. & Hamm, A. 1975. Cerebral hemispheric asymmetry in humans. *Archives of Neurology, 32,* 239-46.

Wahlsten, D. 1979. Some logical fallacies in the classical ethological point of view. *The Behavioral and Brain Sciences, 2,* 48-49.

Wapner, W., Hamby, S. & Gardner, H. 1981. The role of the right hemisphere in the apprehension of complex linguistic materials. *Brain and Language, 14,* 15-33.

Warren, J.M. 1977. Handedness and cerebral dominance in monkeys. In Harnad, Doty, Goldstein, Jaynes & Krauthamer (1977).

Warren, J.M. & Nonneman, A.J. 1976. The search for cerebral dominance in monkeys. *Annals of the New York Academy of Sciences, 280,* 732-44.

Whitaker, H. 1976. A case of the isolation of the language function. In H. Whitaker & H.A. Whitaker (eds.) *Studies in Neurolinguistics, vol 2.* New York: Academic Press.

Whitaker, H.A. 1978. The fallacy of the split brain research. *Cognition and Brain Theory, 2,* 8-10.

Widiger, T.A., Knudson, R.M. & Rorer, L.G. 1980. Convergent and discriminant validity of measures of cognitive styles and abilities. *Journal of Personal and Social Psychology, 39,* 116-29.

Winner, E. & Gardner, H. 1977. The comprehension of metaphor in brain-damaged patients. *Brain, 100,* 717-29.

Witelson, S.F. 1974. Hemispheric specialization for linguistic and nonlinguistic tactual perception using a dichotomous stimulation technique. *Cortex, 10,* 3-17.

Witelson, S.F. 1976. Sex and the single hemisphere: specialization of the right hemisphere for spatial processing. *Science, 193,* 425-27.

Witelson, S.F. 1977a. Developmental dyslexia: two right hemispheres and none left. *Science, 195,* 309-11.

Witelson, S.F. 1977b. Anatomic asymmetry in the temporal lobes: its documentation, phylogenesis, and relationship to functional asymmetry. *Annals of the New York Academy of Sciences, 299,* 328-54.

Witelson, S.F. 1977c. Neural and cognitive correlates of developmental dyslexia: age and sex differences. In C. Shagass, S. Gershon & A.J. Friedhoff (eds.) *Psychopathology and Brain Dysfunction*. New York: Raven Press.

Witelson, S.F. 1977d. Early hemispheric specialization and interhemispheric plasticity: an empirical and theoretical review. In Segalowitz & Gruber (1977a).

Witelson, S.F. 1980. Neuroanatomical asymmetry in left-handers: a review and implications for functional asymmetry. In Herron (1980).

Witelson, S.F. & Pallie, W. 1973. Left hemisphere specialization for language in the newborn: neuroanatomical evidence of asymmetry. *Brain, 96*, 641–47.

Witkin, H.A. & Goodenough, D.R. 1977. Field dependence and interpersonal behavior. *Psychological Bulletin, 84*, 661–89.

Wittig, M.A. & Peterson, A.C. (eds.) 1979. *Sex-Related Differences in Cognitive Functioning*. New York: Academic Press.

Wood, C., Goff, W. & Day, R. 1971. Auditory evoked potentials during speech perception. *Science, 173*, 1248–51.

Wood, F. (ed.) 1980. Noninvasive blood flow studies. *Brain and Language, 9* (1).

Wood, F., Stump, D., McKeehan, A., Sheldon, S. & Proctor, J. 1980. Patterns of regional cerebral blood flow during attempted reading aloud by stutterers both on and off haloperidol medication: evidence for inadequate left frontal activation during stuttering. *Brain and Language, 9*, 141–44.

Wyke, M. 1971. The effects of brain lesions on the learning performance of a bimanual co-ordination task. *Cortex, 7*, 59–72.

Yakovlev, P.I. & Lecours, A.-R. 1967. The myelogenetic cycles of regional maturation in the brain. In A. Minkowski (ed.) *Regional Development of the Brain in Early Life*. Oxford: Blackwell.

Yamadori, A. 1975. Ideogram reading in alexia. *Brain, 98*, 231–38.

Yeni-Komshian, G.H. & Benson, D.A. 1976. Anatomical study of cerebral asymmetry in the temporal lobe of humans, chimpanzee and rhesus monkeys. *Science, 192*, 387–89.

Young, G. 1977. Manual specialization in infancy: implication for lateralization of brain function. In Segalowitz & Gruber (1977a).

Young, G., Corter, C., Segalowitz, S.J. & Trehub, S. (eds.) in press. *Manual Specialization and the Developing Brain: Longitudinal Research.* New York: Academic Press.

Zaidel, D. & Sperry, R.W. 1973. Performance on the Raven's colored progressive matrices test by subjects with cerebral commissurotomy. *Cortex, 9,* 34–39.

Zaidel, E. 1977. Unilateral auditory language comprehension on the Token Test following cerebral commissurotomy and hemispherectomy. *Neuropsychologia, 15,* 1–18.

Zaidel, E. 1979. The split and half brains as models of congenita language disability. In C.L. Ludlow & M.E. Doran-Quine (eds.) *The Neurological Bases of Language Disorders in Children: Methods and Directions for Research.* Bethesda, MD: NINCDS Monograph Series.

Zajonc, R.B. 1980. Feeling and thinking: preferences need no inferences. *American Psychologist, 35,* 151–75.

Zoccolotti, P. & Oltman, P.K. 1978. Field dependence and lateralization of verbal and configurational processing. *Cortex, 14,* 155–68.

Zoccolotti, P., Passafiume, D. & Pizzamiglio, L. 1979. Hemispheric superiorities on a unilateral tactile test: relationship to cognitive dimensions. *Perceptual and Motor Skills, 49,* 735–42.

Zurif, E. & Bryden, M.P. 1969. Familial handedness and left-right differences in auditory and visual perception. *Neuropsychologia, 7,* 179–88.

Zurif, E. & Caramazza, A. 1976. Psycholinguistic structures in aphasia: studies in syntax and semantics. In H. Whitaker & H.A. Whitaker (eds.) *Studies in Neurolinguistics,* vol 1. New York: Academic Press.

Zurif, E. & Mendelsohn, M. 1972. Hemispheric specialization for the perception of speech sounds: the influence of intonation and structure. *Perception and Psychophysics, 11,* 329–32.

Zurif, E. & Ramier, A. 1972. Some effects of unilateral brain damage on the perception of dichotically presented phoneme sequences and digits. *Neuropsychologia, 10,* 103–10.

Zurif, E. & Sait, P. 1970. The role of syntax in dichotic listening. *Neuropsychologia, 8,* 239–44.

Index

Abramson, A.S., 198
Abstract vs. concrete words, 90–92
Ades, A.E., 95
AER, *see* Average evoked response
Affective psychosis, 216–18
Age:
  increase in lateralization with, 109–12
  and left-handedness, 142
  plasticity and, 112–14
  type of lateralization and, 111
  See also Child development
Agenesis of corpus callosum, 52
Agnosia(s), 18, 20, 30–34
  auditory, 31–33
  facial (prosopagnosia), 19, 31
  visual, 30–31
Aitken, L.M., 83
Ajuriaguerra, J., 156
Alajouanine, T., 43
Albert, Martin L., 38, 42–44, 124, 157
"Alien hand" syndrome, 48, 54
Allard, F., 169–70
Alpha waves, 77–78, 86
  hypnotic susceptibility and, 179
  and musical activity, 98
Amadeo, M., 220
Ambidexterity, 142
  and autism, 203
  and learning disorders, 149, 166, 167
American Indian signs, 92
American Sign Language (ASL), 153–54
Ames, Louise, 117, 118, 124
Analytic/holistic dichotomy, 196–98, 219
Andreae, J.H., 15
Andrews, R.J., 157
Animals, lateralization in, 126–31
Anisfeld, M., 157
Annett, M., 156, 157
Anoxia and left-handedness, 149–50
Anterior aphasia, 21
  See also Broca's aphasia
Anterior (frontal) area and speech planning
    and organizing, 27, 41
Apes, lateralization in, 126–28, 131
Aphasia(s), 18, 20–27, 33–34, 85, 89–90
  bilingualism and, 155–56
  Broca's, 8–10, 21, 22, 24, 25, 27, 37, 90, 155,
    195
  in children, 109–10
  conduction, 22, 24
  in deaf subjects, 154
  degree of, after left-hemisphere damage,
    143, 159
  global, 23, 24, 26
  and humor, 40

and intelligence, 27
  intonation in, 37–39
  isolation syndrome, 22–24
  and Japanese writing systems, 91–92, 121–22
  main types of, reviewed, 21–25
  and metaphor, 39–40
  and musical skills, 32–33
  reading in, 91–92
  semantic, 41
  and speech acts, 39
  surgery on left vs. right hemisphere and
    (table), 24
  and tests for language dominance, 26–27
  transcortical motor, 22, 24
  transcortical sensory, 22, 24
  Wernicke's, 9, 10, 21–22, 24, 25, 32–33,
    90, 155
  women vs. men and incidence of, 159
Apraxia(s), 18, 20, 27–30, 33–34
  constructional, 28–29
  dressing, 29
Arbuckle, T.Y., 96
Archibald, Y., 43, 138
Armstrong, D., 123
Arndt, Stephen, 174–75, 183
Arnold, A.P., 171
Articulation, place of, 189, 193
Artifacts, 225–30
  in dichotic listening procedure, 226–27
  in visual half-field technique, 227–29
Artistic ability in autism, 202, 203
Artists
  vs. lawyers, 174–75
  vs. nonartists, and hand preference, 151
Ashton, R., 94–95
ASL (American Sign Language), 153–54
Assal, G., 43
Association areas of brain, 11
Atomists, 181
Auditory agnosia, 31–33
Auditory effects
  dominance for, 97–100
  See also Dichotic listening task
Austin, J.L., 44
Autism, 59, 186 201–2
Average evoked response, (AER), 73–78
  and grammar processing, 90
  and lateralization in newborns, 115
  and voice onset time, 191
Axon, definition of, 5–6

Babbling, 132
Baer, D., 43
Bain, J.D., 95
Bakan, Paul, 138, 149, 157, 180, 183, 211

Bandwidth of speech, 189–91, 193
Barerra, M.E., 116–17, 124
Barsley, M., 138
Battison, R., 157
Beale, I.L., 137, 138, 156, 172, 210
Bebout, L.J., 95, 199
"Belle indifférence," 215–16
Benson, D.A., 127, 136
Benson, D.F., 43, 95
Benton, A.L., 42, 43, 94
Berent, S., 183
Berger, Dale, 174–75, 183
Berlin, C.I., 84, 123, 170
Berlin, H.L., 123, 170
Berlucchi, G., 84, 106
Bernstein, L., 43
Bertoloni, G., 84
Best, C.T., 124
Beta waves, 77–78
Bever, Tom G., 197, 199, 230, 233
Bigelow, L.B., 220–21
Bilingualism, 155–56, 215
Biological reductionism, 235–37
Birds, evidence for lateralization in, 129, 131, 161
Birth stress and left-handedness, 149–51
Blackman, S., 183
Blackstock, E.G., 211
Blakemore, C., 84
Blood flow patterns, *see* Cerebral blood flow
Blumstein, S.E., 95, 96, 105, 124, 233
Bogen, G.M., 60, 137
Bogen, Joseph E., 15, 43, 48, 54, 59, 60, 137, 209, 211
Borowy, T., 171
Bower, T.G.R., 123
Bowers, D., 84
Bowers, K., 183
Bradshaw, J.L., 95, 157
Bragdon, H.R., 84
Brain damage
  early, and lateralization, 144, 152–53
  unilateral, 19–44
    in agnosias, 20, 30–34
    in aphasias, 20–27, 33–34
    in apraxias, 20, 27–30, 33–34
    diagnostic problems, 33–34
    in hemi-spatial neglect, 33
    and language functions, 36–41
    recovery of function after, 34–36
    summary of clinical findings on, 41–42
  See also Recovery of brain function; Split-brain patients
Brain-mind mapping, 234–36
Branff, D., 220
Brann, A.W., 157
Bresson, François, 118, 124, 137
Brinkman, J., 84

Brizzolara, D., 84
Broca, Paul, 8, 18, 145
Broca's aphasia, 8–10, 21, 22, 24, 25, 27, 37, 90, 155, 195
Broca's area, 8, 31, 37
Brown, R.M., 171
Brown, Thomas, 212
Brown, Warren S., 77, 84, 95
Bruce, Lewis C., 215
Bruder, G.E., 220
Bryden, M. Phil, 70, 71, 84, 101, 106, 148, 156, 157, 170–72, 183, 221, 233
Buchsbaum, B., 84
Buchtel, H.A., 84
Buffrey, A.W.H., 171
Butters, N., 123

Cain, D.P., 136
Calculation ability, 41
Caltagirone, C., 198
Cameron, Ralph F., 121, 124, 157
Campanella, D., 96
Capitani, E., 106
Caplan, P., 124
Capra, F., 184
Caramazza, A., 42, 44, 95
Carey, Susan, 93, 96
Carmada, R., 106
Carmon, A., 105, 137–38
Castro-Caldas, A., 157
Catastrophic reaction, 215
CBF, *see* Cerebral blood flow
Cell body, definition of, 5–6
Cerebral blood flow (CBF), 78–80, 83
  handedness and, 134–35, 148–49
  personality type and, 175
  and stuttering, 201
Cerebral cortex:
  definition of, 6
  plasticity and, 113–14
Cerebral hemispheres:
  asymmetries in animals, 126–30
  definition of, 6
  in developing child, *see* Child development
  equipotentiality of, 114–15
  evolutionary advantages of lateralization of, 131–36
  four lobes of, described, 6, 7
  homologous areas in, 10, 36, 37
  individual differences in, *see* Individual differences
  lateralization for linguistic functions, 85–96
  lateralization measurement techniques, 63–82, 225–33
  lateralization for nonlinguistic functions, 97–106
  physical asymmetries of, 10, 18, 122, 126–28
  popular view of specialization of, 57, 197, 206

Cerebral hemispheres, *Cont'd.*
psychodynamic processes and, 203–6,
212–21
relative strength of inter- and intrahemispheric connections, 56
reorganization of function and, 35–36
separation of, *see* Split-brain patients
specific mental conditions and lateralization
of, 200–11
theories of lateralization of, summarized,
187–99
cognitive style, 196–98
fine motor and perceptual planning,
194–96
speech processing, 188–94
unilateral damage to, *see* Unilateral brain
damage
See also Cognitive style; Left hemisphere;
Right hemisphere; Verbal/visual-
spatial dichotomy
Cerebrum, definition of, 6
Chapman, J.A., 84
Chapman, J.S., 124
Chapman, R.M., 84
Chiarello, Robert J., 199, 230, 233
Child development, 109–24
age and degree of asymmetry, 109–12
anatomical asymmetries and, 122
asymmetry at birth, 115–17, 119–23, 198
experience and lateralization in, 119–22
handedness in, 117–19
hemispheric equipotentiality for language,
114–15
lateralization and plasticity in, 112–14
and right hemisphere dominance for
emotions, 219–20
type of lateralization in child vs. adult, 111
Children:
and humor, 40
and metaphor, 39
Chinese ideograms, 169
Choo, G., 84, 183
Chu, J., 105
Cicone, M., 44, 220
Clarke, E., 12–15, 94
Clarke, R., 124, 171
Clarkson, D., 105
Cognitive style, 49, 50
cultural differences and, 180
field dependence and, 175–78
of lawyers vs. artists, 174–75
men vs. women and, 163–65
theory of, summarized, 196–98
See also Hemisphericity; Verbal/visual-
spatial dichotomy
Cohen, B.D., 183
Cohen, G., 84, 199

Cohen, R.A., 184
Colby, K.M., 211
Collins, R.L., 157
Color perception, 104
Cometa, M.S., 44
Commissures:
definition of, 45, 53
See also Corpus callosum
Commissurotomy, 45
complete vs. partial, 53, 58
See also Split-brain patients
Competence as aspect of lateralization, 82
Complementarity, 153, 236
Comprehension of speech, 8, 20–22, 24, 38
See also Wernicke's aphasia
Conceptual disruption, right-hemisphere
damage and, 40–41
Concrete vs. abstract words, 90–92
Concurrent manual tasks, 81
Conduction aphasia, 22, 24
Conflict reduction, brain specialization and, 133
Consciousness, 180, 212–13
altered states of, 203–6
See also Unconscious
Constructional apraxia, 28–29
Contralateral pathways, 66–68
Cook, J., 84
Cooper, F., 95
Cooper, W.E., 96, 105
Corballis, Michael C., 124, 134, 135, 137, 138,
156, 172, 210
Coren, Stanley, 124, 137, 142, 156, 157, 172
Corpus callosum, 69
agenesis of, 52
cutting of, *see* Commissurotomy; Split-
brain patients
definition of, 6, 7
in hearing, 66–68
myelination of, 59
Correlation coefficient, 77
Corter, C., 124
Cortex, *see* Cerebral cortex
Cox, G.B., 204, 211
Cox, P.W., 183
Crawford, H.T., 170–71
Cross-cueing in split-brain patients, 50–52
Crossed eye-dominance and dyslexia, 167
Crovitz, H.F., 156
"Crowding" hypothesis, 132, 133, 150–51, 166,
172
Crowne, D., 43
Culebras, A., 127
Cullen, J.K., Jr., 84
Currier, R.D., 124, 157
Curry, F., 105
Curtiss, S., 157
Cutting, J.E., 198, 199

Dabbs, James M., 84, 175, 183
Dalrymple, A., 124
Damasio, A.R., 157, 211
Danly, M., 44
Darwin, C.J., 95, 198
Davidoff, J., 84
Davidson, R.J., 105, 106
Dawson, G., 156, 211
Dawson, J.L.M.B., 183
Day, R., 84
de Schonen, S., 124, 137
Deaf, lateralization in, 153-54, 194
DeAgostini, M., 238
Debes, J.L., 184
Dee, H., 106
DeLuca, D., 44
Denckla, M.B., 84
Dendrites:
    and brain plasticity, 113-14
    definition of, 5-6
Denenberg, Victor H., 130, 137
Dennis, Maureen, 43, 44, 60, 114-15,
    123, 172
Depression, 215-18
Descartes, Rene, 11, 181
Dewey, J., 238
Dewhurst, K., 12-15, 94
Dewson, J.H., III, 137
Diamond, R., 220
Dichotic listening task, 56, 66-69, 82, 93-94
    artifacts in, 226-27
    and bilingualism, 155
    with children, 111, 112, 115-16
    and dominance for emotions, 101-2
    and dominance for music, 99-100
    grammatical functions and, 90
    and hypnosis, 204-5
    with lefthanders, 144
    male-female comparison, 165
    and maturation rate of girls vs. boys, 162
    with monkeys, 129
    Navajo-Anglo comparison, 182-83
    and nonverbal vocal sounds, 97-98
    and speech processing, 87-89, 188, 193
Dichhaptic task, 71-73
    with dyslexics, 168-69
Dichotomies, 196-98, 200, 208-10
    listed, 209
    See also Verbal/visual-spatial dichotomy
Differences, individual, see Individual
    differences
Diffuse/focal dichotomy, 198
Dimond, S.J., 220
Dingwall, W.O., 43
Direct measures, definition of, 229
Dirkes, M.A., 211
Doehring, D., 172

Dominance:
    definition of, 36, 83
    mixed, 151
    See also Language, (left) dominance for;
        Left hemisphere; Right hemisphere
Dorman, M.F., 171
Double dissociation, 20
Doubleday, D.N., 105
Dreaming, 204-6
Dressing apraxia, 29
Dumas, R., 183
Duncan, P., 124, 157
Dynamic aphasia, see Transcortical motor
    aphasia
Dynamic psychology, 186
Dyslexia, 59, 166-69, 200-1

Ear preference, 119, 120
Ears, see Dichotic listening task
ECT and field dependence, 176-78
Edmonston, W.E., 105
Education, right hemisphere and, 206-8, 210
EEG, see Electroencephalograph
Efron, R., 199
Ehrichman, H., 84, 95, 183
Eimas, Peter D., 110-11, 123, 198
Electro-convulsive therapy (ECT) and field
    dependence, 177-78
Electrodermal measurements of lateralization,
    80
Electroencephalograph (EEG), 73-78, 83,
    89, 102
    extension of response and, 214
    in schizophrenia vs. affective psychosis,
    216-17
    See also Alpha waves; Average evoked
        response
Embedded-figure task, 176-77
Emotional vs. nonemotional words, 91, 101-2
Emotions, 41-42, 101-2, 213-14
    right hemisphere and, 101-2, 214-16, 218-20
    in rats, 129-30
    sex differences and, 164
    visual half-field technique and, 69-71, 82,
    101
Encoded speech, 88-89, 189, 191
Engle (author), 137
Entus, Anne Kasman, 115-16, 124
Environment, see Heredity-environment
    debate
Epilepsy, 20, 45, 52, 57-58
Equipotentiality, hemispheric, 114-15
Erikson, Eric H., 221
Eson, M.E., 44
Evans, E.A., 157
Evans, F.J., 183

Evans, G.W., 170
Evoked response
average, *see* Average evoked response (AER)
definition of, 73-75
Evolution, advantages of lateralization in, 131-36
Eye movements, *see* Lateral eye movements (LEM)
Eye preference, 119, 120
and dyslexia, 151, 167
Experience
effect on lateralization of, 119-22
See also Cognitive style; Heredity-environment debate

Facial agnosia (prospagnosia), 19, 31
Facial recognition, 19, 34, 49-50, 52, 58, 102-4, 197
visual half-field technique, 69-71, 82, 101, 102
Familial sinistrality, 145
Fedio, P., 84
Feelings, *see* Emotions
Fennell, E B., 84, 157
Ferro, J.M., 157
Field dependence, 175-78
sex differences and, 163
Figurative language, *see* Metaphor
Fincham, R.W., 43
Fine motor planning, 194-96
Fischer (author), 127
Fischer, F.W., 172
Fischler, I., 157
Flamm, L., 44
Flor-Henry, Pierre, 217, 220, 221
Florian, V.A., 157
Fluent aphasia, 216
See also Werniche's aphasia
Focal/diffuse dichotomy, 198
Folb, S., 105
Foldi, N.S., 44, 220
Fontenot, D., 106
Foot preference, 119, 120
Forant transitions, 188-91, 193
Franzini, C., 106
Frediani, A.W., 170
Freeman, R.B., 124
Freud, Sigmund, 205, 213
"Freudian slips", 55
Frisch, H.L., 171
Fritsch, Gustav Theodor, 8, 18
Fromkin, V.A., 95
Frumkin, L.R., 204, 211
Frontal (anterior) area and speech planning and organizing, 27, 41
Frontal aphasia, 21
See also Broca's aphasia

Frontal lobe:
definition of, 6, 7
reorganization of, after damage, 35
Fuller, P., 211
Futer, D., 43

Gainotti, G., 198, 220
Galaburda, A.M., 136
Galin, David, 60, 77-78, 84, 86, 94, 183, 184, 211, 212-13, 220
Galkin, T.W., 170, 171
Gall, Franz, 7-8
Garbanati, J., 137
Gardiner, M.F., 124, 184
Gardner, Howard, 40, 42-44, 220
Garvin (author), 65
Gatzoyas, A., 157
Gazzaniga, Michael S., 1, 50, 51, 53, 55, 59, 60, 84, 106, 199, 211, 214, 220
Geffner, D.S., 171
General activation, 80-81
Genessee, F., 124
Geschwind, Norman, 15, 23, 43, 83, 126-27, 136
Gesell, Arnold, 117, 118, 124
Gestural systems, 135-36
Giannitrapani, D., 221
Gilbert, C., 157
Glanville, B.B., 124
Glassman, R.B., 15
Glencross, D.J., 84
Global aphasia, 23, 24, 26
Godfrey, J., 95
Goebel, R., 171
Goff, W., 84
Goldman, P.S., 170, 171
Goldman, R.D., 137, 157
Goldstein, K., 183
Goldstein, M.H., Jr., 83
Gombos, G.M., 137-38
Goodenough, D.R., 183
Goodglass, H., 42, 43, 105
Gordon, H.W., 43, 105, 199, 210, 233
Gordon, J., 44
Gott, P.S., 60
Grammar, *see* Syntax
Gray, C., 220
Gray, J.A., 171
Greenough, W.T., 211
Greenwood, P., 211
Grey matter, *see* Cerebral cortex
Grossman, Murray, 93, 96
Grosso, J.T., 157
Gruber, F.A., 84, 138, 199, 233
Gruzelier, J., 220, 221
Gur, R.C., 183, 184
Gur, Raquel E., 175, 183, 184, 220

Haapanen, R., 211
Haerer, A.F., 124, 157
Hakansson, K., 137-38, 157
Hall, J.L., II, 83
Hallucinations, 182-83
Halverson, H., 124
Hamby, S., 44
Hamilton, C.R., 137
Hamm, A., 124, 171
Handedness, 8, 56, 132-36, 141-51
  in animals, 130, 136
  artists vs. nonartists and, 151
  culture and, 119, 134, 142
  and dominance for language, 8, 20, 132
  early brain damage and language repre-
    sentation, 152
  evolutionary advantages of, 134-35
  genetic explanations for, 145-48
  heredity and, 119, 133
  in individual development, 117-20
  inverted writing posture and, 145-48
  and lateralization, 143-45
  nongenetic explanations for, 148-50
  and spatial skills, 132
  See also Ambidexterity; Left-handedness;
    Right-handedness
Handel, A.B., 199
Hansson, P., 95, 96, 199
"Hard-wiring" vs. "soft-wiring" of brain,
  234-35
Hardyck, Curtis, 137, 150, 156, 157, 211
Harnad, S.R., 138
Harris, A.J., 156
Harris, L.J., 138, 156, 169, 170
Harshman, R.A., 170
HAS (high amplitude sucking), 115-16
Hatta, T., 95
Haynes, W.O., 84
Hearing, see Dichotic listening task
Hebrew, writing posture hypotheses and,
  147-48
Hécaen, Henri, 35, 36, 42, 43, 156, 157, 238
Heeschen, C., 44, 93-94, 96
Heilman, Ken M., 1-2, 42, 44, 92, 96, 220
Helm, Nancy A., 38, 44
Hemiparesis, 114-15
Hemi-spatial neglect syndrome, 33
Hemispheres, see Cerebral hemispheres
Hemisphericity, 173-84
  cultural differences and, 180-83
  definition of, 173-74
  field dependence and, 178
  hypnotic susceptibility and, 179-80
  television and, 180
  personality and, 174-75
Hendrick, E.B., 123
Hepburn, M.J., 184

Heredity-environment debate:
  degree of lateralization at birth, 115-17,
    119-23, 198
  and handedness, 119, 133
Hermalin, B., 84, 124
Herron, J., 60, 157
Hicks, E., 84
Hicks, R.A., 157
High amplitude sucking (HAS), 115-16
Hilgard, J.R., 183
Hillyard, Stephen, 51, 60
Hines, D., 95
Hiscock, M., 84, 94-95, 112, 123
Hitzig, Edward, 8, 18
Hochberg, F.H., 127
Hochberg, I., 171
Hoemann, H.W., 157
Hoffman, C., 183
Hoffman, H.J., 123
Holism, 7, 8, 11
  on language, 23
Holistic/analytic dichotomy, 196-98, 219
Homologous areas, 37
  definition of, 10
  in regained function, 36
Hoppe, Klaus D., 205-6, 211
Hormones and sex differences in lateralization,
  160-61
Hughes, L.F., 123, 170
Huling, M.D., 172
Humor; aphasics vs. right brain-damaged and,
  40, 42
Humphrey, M.E., 211
Hunt, L., 184
Hurtig, R.R., 199
Huttenlocher, P.R., 123
Huws, D., 220
Hynd, G.W., 184
Hypnosis, 55, 179-80, 203-5, 210
Hysterical paralysis, 55, 213

Illocutionary force, 39
Imagery, see Verbal/visual-spatial dichotomy
Indifference reactions, 215-16
Individual differences, 139-84, 230-31, 235
  in brain organization, 141-57
    early experiences, 153-56
    effects of early brain damage, 152-53
    handedness, 141-57
  cause-effect problem and, 236-37
  in degree of asymmetry, 158-72
    and reading disability, 166-69
    sex and, 158-66
  diagnosis in brain damage and, 34
  in hemisphericity, 173-84
    artists vs. lawyers, 174-75
    cultural factors, 180-83

Individual differences, *Cont'd.*
    field dependence, 175-78
    hypnotic susceptibility, 179-80
    television, 180
    in split-brain patients, 53, 57-58
Inertia, concurrent manual tasks and, 81
Inglis, J., 170
Ingram, D., 124
Ingvar, D.H., 79, 84
Intelligence, aphasia and, 27
Interactive vs. linear mind-brain model, 236-37
Intonation, 37-39, 87, 93, 99, 101
Ipsilateral pathways, 66, 68
Isaacson, R.L., 157
Isolation from language, 154-55
Isolation of speech area (aphasic syndrome), 22-24
Itoh, M., 95

Jackendoff, R., 43
Jacklin, C.N., 169, 171
Jackson, John Hughlings, 10, 15, 85, 165
Jacobson, M.J., 43
Japanese writing systems, 91-92, 121-22, 194
Jaynes, Julian, 102, 103, 106, 182, 184
Jensen, A.R., 172
John, E.R., 220
Johnson, D.D., 172
Johnson, O., 94-95
Johnstone, J., 60
Jones, M.B., 157
Jones, R.K., 210
Jung, Carl Gustav, 213
Jurgens, R., 93-94, 96
Juscyk, P., 123, 198

Kagan, S., 183
Kana writing system, 91-92
Kanji writing system, 91-92, 194
Kaplan, C.D., 184
Kaplan, E., 43
Kaplan, R., 137
Kaprinis, G., 157
Katz (author), 172
Katz, A.N., 211
Kemper, T.L., 136
Kertesz, A., 25, 43, 170
Kimura, Doreen, 28, 43, 67, 83, 84, 87-88, 94-95, 99, 105, 106, 138, 156, 157, 170, 195, 199, 226, 233
King, F.L., 105
Kinsbourne, Marcel, 44, 60, 84, 94-95, 112, 123, 124, 132-33, 137, 156, 233
Kitchener, R.F., 238
Knowledge, disorders of, *see* Agnosia(s)
Knudson, R.M., 183
Kobayashi, Y., 95

Kohn, B., 123, 172
Kolb, B., 43
Kotik, Bella, 155, 157
Kozma, A., 94-95
Krashen, S.D., 123, 170
Krech, D., 15
Kuhl, P.K., 198
Kuypers, H.G.J.M., 84

Lackner, J., 106
Lake, D., 157, 170
Lancaster, J., 138
Lane, H., 157
Language, 8-10, 34, 85-96
    bilingualism, 155-56, 215
    components of, *see* Phonology; Semantics; Syntax; Pragmatics of language
    early brain damage and speech representation, 152
    evolutionary origins of, 9, 135-36
    hemispheric equipotentiality for, 114-15
    individual development of lateralization for, 109-12, 115-17, 122-23
    isolation from, 154-55
    (left) dominance for, 8-10, 18, 20, 23-24, 27-28, 34, 36, 37, 41, 48, 49, 85-86, 88-94, 100
        babbling and, 132
        and dyslexia, 166-68
        handedness and, 132, 143-45, 150-52
        Navajo-Anglo comparison, 182-83
        phonology, 37, 86-89, 188-94
        physical asymmetries and, 126-28
        planning function as basis for, 194-95
        pragmatics, 87, 93-94
        semantics, 37, 87, 90-92
        social clan and, 171
        syntax, 37, 48-49, 87, 89-90, 93-94
        testing for, 26-27
        time discrimination, 100, 194
        in women vs. men, 159, 162, 164
    literacy and brain organization, 121, 153
    location of centers of, 8-10, 26
    loss of, *see* Aphasia
    planning and organizing of, 26-27, 41, 195-96
    prelinguistic skills, 110-11, 115-17, 189, 191
    right hemisphere and, 10, 36-42, 48-49, 89-94, 144, 153-56
    in split-brain patients, 48-49, 57
    in schizophrenia, 216
    testing for dominance, 26-27
    See also Reading; Verbal/visual-spatial dichotomy; Writing
Lansdell, H., 170, 171
Lansky, L.M., 157
Lassen, N.A., 84

Lateral eye movements (LEMs), 80-81, 86, 101
and hypnotizability, 180
in lefthanders, 144
Lateralization:
definition of, 82-83
See also Cerebral hemispheres; Verbal/visual-spatial dichotomy
Lavy, S., 105
Lawson, J.S., 170
Lawson, N.C., 157
Lawyers vs. artists, 174-75
Learning disorders:
left-handedness and, 149, 166-67
See also Dyslexia
Lecours, A.R., 60
Lederman, S.J., 95, 199
LeDoux, Joseph, 50, 53, 55, 59, 60, 84, 106, 214, 220
Left-handedness, 136, 138
and autism, 203
birth stress and, 149-50
definition of, 142
evolutionary advantages of, 135
generic explanations for, 145-48
incidence of, 141-42
and learning disorders, 149, 166-67
and left-lateralization for language, 132
nongenetic explanations for, 148-52
See also Handedness
Left hemisphere:
and apraxia, 27-30
and auditory agnosia, 31-33
ECT and, 177-78
intellectual strengths of, in split-brain patients, 48-50
and language, *see* Language, (left) dominance for
and prelinguistic skills, 115
and visual agnosia, 31
See also Cerebral hemispheres; Verbal/visual-spatial dichotomy
LeMay, Marjorie, 126-27, 136
Lempert, H., 137
LEMs, *see* Lateral eye movements
Lenneberg, E.H., 43, 123
Lerner, R.M., 238
Lesk, D., 25
Levenson, R., 124
Livitsky, W., 15
Levy, Jerre, 84, 131-33, 137, 145-47, 157, 165-66, 170-72
Ley, Robert S., 56, 60, 70, 71, 84, 91, 95, 101-2, 104, 106, 220, 221
Liberman, A., 95
Liberman, I.Y., 172
Lieberman, P., 138
Linden, E., 137

Linear vs. interactive mind-brain model, 236-37
Ling, P.K. 44
Lishman, W.A., 157
Lisker, L., 198
Literacy and lateralization, 121, 153
Lloyd, B., 171
Localizationism, 7-8, 10-14
on language, 8, 23
and reorganization of function, 36
Lomas, J., 84, 94-95
Lovett, M., 123
Lowe-Bell, L.F., 123, 170
Luria, Alexandr R., 22, 41, 43, 156, 199

McCabe, P., 25
Maccoby, E.E., 169, 171
McCraig, J.W., 84
McDonald, F.J., 184
McDonald, H., 184
McFarland, K., 94-95
McFarland, M.L., 95
McGee, M.G., 171, 172
McGhee, M.G., 44
McGlone, Jeanette, 159, 170, 171
McKeehan, A., 210
McKeever, W.F., 157, 172, 184, 210
McMeekan, E., 157
McNeil, M.R., 84
Maer, F., 106
Manual tasks, concurrent, 81
Marcel, T., 172
Marsh, J.T., 77, 84, 95
Marshalek, B., 183
Marshall, J., 171
Marzi, C., 84, 106
Mason, J.W., 171
Matthew, Gospel of, 45
Maturation and sex differences in lateralization, 161-62
Maurer, R.G., 211
Maury, L., 124, 137
Mavlov, Ludmil, 100, 105
Meaning, *see* Semantics
Measurement techniques, 63-82, 225-33
artifacts in, 225-30
direct, definition of, 229
relative, 231-33
See also specific procedures
Mebert, C.J., 151, 157
Melodic intonation therapy, 38-39
Melodic skills, 38, 41-42, 99
Mendelsohn, M., 95
Mesulam, M.M., 44, 220
Metaphor, 39-40
Miceli, G., 198
Michel (author), 44
Miller, J.D., 198

Mills, L., 105, 199
Milner, Brenda, 32, 43, 99-100, 105, 143-44, 152, 156, 220
Mind, 6-7, 11, 12
 mapping of, onto brain, 234-36
 sociology of, 55, 59, 214
 of split-brain patients vs. normals, 45, 53-57
Mitchell, D., 84
Mitchell, G.F., 151, 157
Mixed dominance, 151
Molfese, Dennis L., 84, 95, 115, 123, 124, 191-93, 198
Molfese, V.J., 123, 124
Monkeys, lateralization in, 126-29, 131
Monzon-Montes, A., 238
Moore, W.H., Jr., 84
Morgan, A., 183, 184
Morgan, M.J., 137
Mori, K., 95
Morrell, M., 170
Moscovitch, Morris, 44, 103, 106, 123, 157
Mosidge, V.M., 43
Moss, H., 171
Motor aphasia, 21
 See also Broca's aphasia
Movements:
 disturbances of, see Apraxia(s)
 planning of, 26-27, 195
Munk, H., 30
Musical skills, 31-33, 98-101
 handedness and, 151
 in HAS procedure, 115-16
Myelination of corpus callosum, 59
Myers, R.E., 56, 60, 157
Myslobodsky, M.S., 84

Nachshon, I., 105, 156
"Nadia" (autistic girl), 202, 203
Nagylaki, T., 157
Nakell, L., 60
Nash, J., 171
Nasrallah (author), 221
Nature vs. nurture, see Heredity-environment debate
Navajo-Anglo comparison for speech lateralization, 182-83
Naylor, H., 210
Nebes, R.D., 59
Neglect syndrome, hemi-spatial, 33
Neisser, U., 238
Neonatal lateralization, 115-17, 119-23, 198
Netley, C., 44
Neurons:
 and brain plasticity, 113-14
 definition of, 5-6
 recovery from damage, 34-35
 subcortical, 6

Neuropsychology, development of, 6-12
Newcombe, F., 137
Nonneman, A.J., 137
Nottebohm, Fernando, 129, 137, 161, 171

Obler, L., 157
O'Brien, B., 184
Occipital lobe:
 definition of, 6, 7
 and reading, 35
O'Connor, N., 84, 124
Ojemann, G.A., 43
Oldfield, R.C., 156, 157
Olds, J., 106
Oltman, P.K., 183
Onset time, 189, 191-93
Organizing of language, 26-27, 41, 195-96
Orr, C., 183, 232, 233
Ornstein, Robert, 77-78, 84, 86, 94, 183, 184
Orton, Samuel, 166-68, 172, 200-1, 210

"P.S." (split-brain subject), 52, 54, 58
Paivio, A., 106
Palermo, D.S., 124
Pallie, W., 124
Paradis, Michael, 124, 155-57
Paredes, J.A., 184
Park, S., 96
Parkinson, C., 211
Parsons, J., 169, 171
Passafiume, D., 183
Pavlidis, G., 172, 233
Payer-Rigo, P., 198
PCA (principal components analysis), 76
Parietal lobe, definition of, 6, 7
Participation as aspect of lateralization, 83
Paw preference, 130
Pelligrini, R.J., 157
Penfield, W., 8, 9, 43
Pergament, L., 157
Perseverative errors, 28
Personality:
 of artists vs. lawyers, 174-75
 See also Cognitive style; Hemisphericity
Peters, M., 124
Petersen, A.C., 169, 171
Peterson, J.M., 157
Petrie, B., 124
Petrinovich, L.F., 137, 156, 157
Pettito, L.A., 137
Phoneme, definition of, 86-87
Phonology (sounds), 37, 86-89
 See also Speech sounds
Phrenology, 7-8, 12, 13
Piazza, D.M., 106, 123
Piérant-Le-Bonniec, G., 124, 137
Pineal gland, 11

Pizzamiglio, L., 183
Place of articulation, 189, 193
Planning function, 26-27, 41, 195
Planum temporale, 126-28
Plasticity, 112-14
  See also Recovery of brain function
Poizner, H., 157
Porac, Claire, 124, 137, 142, 156, 157, 172
Poritsky, S., 172
Porter, R.J., 123
Portnoy, Z., 105
Posterior aphasia, see Wernicke's aphasia
Posterior (rear) area and semantic function, 27, 41
Pragmatics of language, 87, 93-94
  See also Intonation; Speech acts
Prelinguistic skills, 110-11, 115-17, 189, 191
Primary process, 205
Primates:
  functional asymmetries in, 128-29
  neuroanatomical asymmetries in, 126-28
Principal components analysis (PCA), 76
Proctor, J., 210
Production of speech, 8, 20-22, 24, 34, 38-39
  See also Broca's aphasia
Profession, choice of, 174-75, 208
Prohovnik, I., 137-38, 157
Prosopagnosia, 19, 31
Provins, K.A., 84
Pryce, I.J., 220
Psalms, 4
Psychic blindness, 30
Psychosis, 216-18
  See also Schizophrenia
Psychotherapy, 55
Puberty, hypothesis of lateralization by, 110

Quadfasel, F.A., 23, 43

Rajan, P., 172
Ramier, A., 95
Rapid eye movement (REM) activity, 205
Rasmussen, Theodore, 143-44, 152, 156
Ratcliffe, G., 137
Rats, evidence for lateralization in, 129-30
Rattok, J., 84
Ravel, Maurice, 32
Ray, W.J., 170
Reading, 91-92
  dyslexia, 59, 166-69, 200-1
  eye preference and problems with, 151
  Japanese writing systems, 91-92, 121-22, 194
  loss of occipital lobe and, 35
Rear (posterior) area and semantic function, 27, 41
Recognition:
  disorders of, see Agnosia(s)
  facial, see Facial recognition

Recovery of brain function, 34-36, 52, 152
  in left-handedness, 143
  physiological, 34-35
  plasticity and, 112-14
  reorganization in, 35-36, 52, 53
  in women vs. men, 159
Reduction, biological, 235-37
Reid, Marylou, 84, 145-47, 157, 170-72
Reisches (author), 44
Relational ideas, 41, 93
Relative measures, use of, 231-33
Relaxation, 210
REM activity, 205
Remington, R., 105, 170
Reorganization, see Recovery of brain function
Repetition in speech, capacity for, 20-22, 24
Rete mirabile, 11
Right-handedness:
  evolutionary choice of, 134-35
  See also Handedness
Right hemisphere, 97-105, 179-83
  and apraxia, 28-30
  cultural differences and, 180-83
  and dreaming, 205
  and dyslexia in girls vs. boys, 168-69
  ECT and, 177-78
  and education, 206-8, 210
  and emotions, 101-2, 214-16, 218-20
  and facial recognition, 19, 34, 49-50, 52, 58, 102-4, 197
  and fine judgments, 195-96
  hypnotic susceptibility and, 179
  importance accorded to, 10, 85, 97, 179
  an individual development, 109, 116-17
  intellectual strengths of, in split-brain patients, 48-50
  and language, 10, 36-42, 48-49, 89-94, 144, 153-56
  and melodic skills, 38, 41-42, 99
  and music, 31-32, 98-101
  and nonverbal vocal sounds, 97-98, 101
  and psychosis, 216-18
  recognition of designs and, 104
  and relaxation, 210
  and spatial skills, 41-42, 49, 50, 109
  television and, 180
  and unconscious, 212-13
  See also Cerebral hemispheres; Verbal/Visual-spatial dichotomy
Rimland, B., 211
Ripley, H.S., 204, 211
Risberg, J., 84, 137-38, 157
Risse, Gail, 53, 60
Rizzolatti, G., 84, 106
Roberts (author), 137
Roberts, L., 8, 9, 43
Robinson, G.M., 105, 199
Robinson, R.G., 137

Rod-and-frame test, 176
Roemer, R.A., 220
Rogers, L., 184
Rollman, G.B., 105, 199
Rorer, L.G., 183
Rosadini, G., 156, 220
Rose, H., 211
Rose, Steven, 211, 235–36, 238
Rosen, J.J., 123
Rosenthal, R., 220–21
Rosenzweig, M.R., 83, 211
Ross, E.D., 44, 220
Ross, Phyllis, 49–50, 60, 103–4, 106, 157, 197,
   199, 229, 233
Rossi, G.F., 156, 220
Rosvold, H.E., 170, 171
Roth, R.S., 220
Rothi, L., 96
Rourke, B.P., 210
Rozin, P., 172
Rubens, A.B., 15, 43, 126
Rudel, R.G., 84
Russell, Bertrand, 184
Russell, I.S., 43

St. James-Roberts, I., 123, 157
Sait, P., 95
Sameroff, A.J., 171
Samuels, J.A., 95
Sasasuma, S., 95
Satz, P., 84, 156, 157
Sauget, J., 156, 157
Saul, R.E., 60
Scammell, R., 220
Scanning, 106
   in dyslexics, 167–68
Schaller, G.B., 137
Schizophrenia, 182, 183, 216–18
Schneider, G.E., 157
Scholes, R.J., 44, 157, 220
Schucard, D.W., 105
Schucard, J.L., 105
Schwartz, G.E., 105, 106
Schwartz, J., 105, 199
Schwartz, M., 157
Scott, S., 184
Scotti, G., 106
Searle, J., 44
Segalowitz, N.S., 95, 96, 199
Segalowitz, S.J., 42, 60, 84, 95, 124, 138, 199,
   228, 232, 233
Segarra, J.M., 23, 43
Seidenberg, L.A., 137
Selfe, L., 202, 211
Selves, 213–14
Semantics (meaning), 37, 87, 90–92
   posterior area and, 27, 41

Semmes, J., 199
Sensory modalities, see Dichotic listening task;
   Touch; Visual half-field technique;
   Visual skills
Seth, G., 124
Sex differences in lateralization, 158–66
   cognitive explanations of, 163–65
   in dyslexics, 168–69
   evidence on, 159–60
   neurophysiological explanations of, 160–62
   and verbal-spatial distinction, 159–62,
   165–66
Shagass, C., 220
Shakespeare, William, 4
Shankweiler, Donald, 88, 95, 157, 172
Shanon, B., 157
Shapiro, B., 44
Shearer, S.L., 220
Shebalin, V.G., 32–33
Sheldon, S., 210
Sherman, G., 137
Shultz, T.R., 44
Sidtis, J.J., 106
Sign language:
   deaf and, 153–54, 194
   in primates, 128, 137
Siqueland, F.R., 123, 198
Silverman, A.J., 183
Silverman, J., 44
Singing skill, 98–99
Sinistrality:
   familial, 145
   See also Left-handedness
Skin conductance, 80
Skinhoj, E., 84
Smith (author), 172
Smith, A., 43
Smith, C., 171
Smith, J.C., 77, 84, 95
Smith, L.C., 157
Smith, M.O., 105
Social clan, lateralization for speech and
   171
Sociology of mind, 55, 59, 214
Sodium amytal, 26
   See also Wada test
"Soft-wiring" vs. "hard-wiring" of brain,
   234–35
Solomon, D.J., 105, 199
Sotsky, R., 172
Soul, 11
Sounds:
   nonverbal, 97–100
   See also Phonology; Speech sounds
Spalten, E., 84
Sparks, Robert, 38, 44, 83
Spatial location, 104

Spatial skills:
 bilateralization for language and, 132, 150-51
 cultural differences and, 181-82
 dyslexia and lateralization of, 168-69
 left-handedness and, 150-51
 right hemisphere dominance for, 41-42, 49, 50, 109
 sex differences and, 159-62, 165-66
 See also Verbal/Visual-spatial dichotomy
Speech, see Language
Speech acts, 39, 87
Speech sounds:
 babies' ability to distinguish, 110-11, 115-17
 processing of, 86-89, 188-94
 See also Dichotic listening test; Phonology
Spellacy, F., 95, 124, 233
Sperry, R.W., 59, 60
Spinnler, H., 106
Split-brain patients, 2, 3, 18, 45-60, 195-96
 adaptation by, 52
 cross-cueing in, 50-52
 dreaming in, 205-6
 individual differences in, 53, 57-58
 intellectual strengths of each hemisphere in, 48-50
 intonation/singing skill and, 99
 language functions in, 48-49, 57
 as model for normals, 54-59
 tactile skills in, 46, 47
 "two minds" of, 45, 53-54
 visual skills in, 46-50, 52, 53
Spreen, O., 43
Springer, S.P., 60
Sprouting, 35
Spurzheim, Johann, 7-8
Steady state vowels, 88
Stein, D.G., 123
Steklis, H.D., 138
Stenslie, C.E., 220
Stewart, C., 84, 233
Stokes, L.P., 170, 171
Stomp, D., 278
Strings, three-word, 93-94
Structured vs. unstructured word strings, 93-94
Studdert-Kennedy, Michael, 88, 95, 157
Stuttering, 201
Subcortex:
 neurons of, 6
 and superior plasticity of child, 113
Sugarman, J.H. 106
Sylvian fissure, 10, 126-28
Symptoms, double dissociation of, 20
Syntax (grammar), 37, 48-49, 87, 89-90, 93-94

Tallal, P., 105, 199
Tanguay, P.E., 105
Tartter, V., 105
Taub, J.M., 105
Taylor, J., 15
Taylor, M.J., 157
Television and hemisphericity, 180
Temporal lobe:
 definition of, 6, 7
 and musical skills, 32, 99-100
 planum temporale of, 126-28
 right-hemisphere electrical stimulation of, 26
TenHouten, W., 184
Terrace, H., 137
Terzian, H., 220
Teuber, H., 106
Thomas, D.G., 105
Time discrimination, 100, 194
Tone onset time, 191
Touch, 46, 64
 dichhaptic task in measuring lateralization of, 71-73, 168-69
 in split-brain patients, 46, 47, 52
Transcortical motor aphasia, 22, 24
Transcortical sensory aphasia, 22, 24
Transitions (speech sounds), 88, 188-91, 193
Trehub, S., 123, 124
Triangulation, 82
Trukese navigators, 181-82
Tsvetkova, L.S., 43
Tucker, D., 170
Tucker, Don M., 217, 220
Turkewitz, Gerald, 49-50, 60, 103-4, 106, 197, 229, 233
"Two-term series" problems, 40-41
Tzavara, A., 157

Umilta, C., 84, 106
Unconscious, 182, 186, 212-13
Unilateral brain damage, see Brain damage, unilateral
Uttal, W.R., 15

Vaid, J., 124
Valenstein, E., 42
Van Deventer, A.D., 157, 172, 210
Van Lancker, D., 95
Vanderplas (author), 65
Vargha-Khadem, F., 124
Verbal environment, 164
Verbal/visual-spatial dichotomy, 41-42, 55, 59, 61, 97-98, 102, 105, 121, 131-32, 236
 cultural differences and, 181-82
 and left-handedness, 150-51
 limitations of, 196-98

Verbal/visual-spatial dichotomy, *Cont'd.*
  women vs. men and, 159-62, 164-66
  See also Cognitive style
Vigorito, J., 123, 198
Visual agnosias, 30-31
Visual environment, 163-64
Visual half-field technique, 69-71, 82, 101, 102, 144
  artifacts in, 227-29
  with deaf subjects, 153-54
  with dyslexics, 168-69
  with lawyers vs. artists, 174-75
Visual skills, 46, 64, 65
  fine judgments and, 195
  right-hemisphere dominance for, 41-42
  in split-brain patients, 46-50, 52, 53
  See also Verbal/visual-spatial dichotomy; Visual half-field technique
Voice onset time, 89, 189, 191-93

Waber, Deborah, 162, 171
Wachtel, P.I., 183
Wada, John A., 26, 124, 136, 171
Wada test, 26, 67, 201, 216
  on early damage and language representation, 152
  on handedness and lateralization, 143, 152
  and musical skills, 32, 98
Wahlsten, D., 211
Walter, D.O., 124
Wapner, W., 44
Warren, J.M., 137
Warrenburg, S., 211
Watson, R.G., 220
Watson, R.T., 1-2, 44, 220
Waveform, definition of, 73
Webster, W.R., 83
Weed, W., 184
Weinberger, A., 95
Weinberger, H., 84

Wernicke, Carl, 10, 18
Wernicke's aphasia, 9, 10, 21-22, 24, 25, 32-33, 90, 155
Wernicke's area, 10, 31, 201
Whishaw, I.Q., 43
Whitaker, H.A., 43, 44, 60, 123
White matter, definition of, 6
Widiger, T.A., 183
Wiegel-Crump, C.A., 123
Wilson, D.H., 60, 211
Winner, Ellen, 40, 44
Witelson, Sandra F., 15, 71, 72, 84, 123, 124, 127, 136, 168-70, 172
Witkin, H.A., 183
Wittig, M.A., 169
Wolfson, S., 96
Wood, C., 84
Wood, F., 84, 210
Word deafness, 31
Words:
  abstract vs. concrete, 90-92
  See also Semantics
Writing, 33
  posture for, handedness and, 145-48
Wyke, M., 43

Yakovlev, P.I., 60
Yamadori, A., 95
Yeni-Komshian, G.H., 127, 136
Yeo, C.H., 43
Young, G., 124
Yozawitz, A., 220
Yutzey, D.A., 137

Zaidel, D., 59, 60
Zajonc, R.B., 220
Zangwill, O.L., 211
Zener, K., 156
Zoccolotti, P., 183
Zurif, E.B., 42, 44, 95, 156, 157

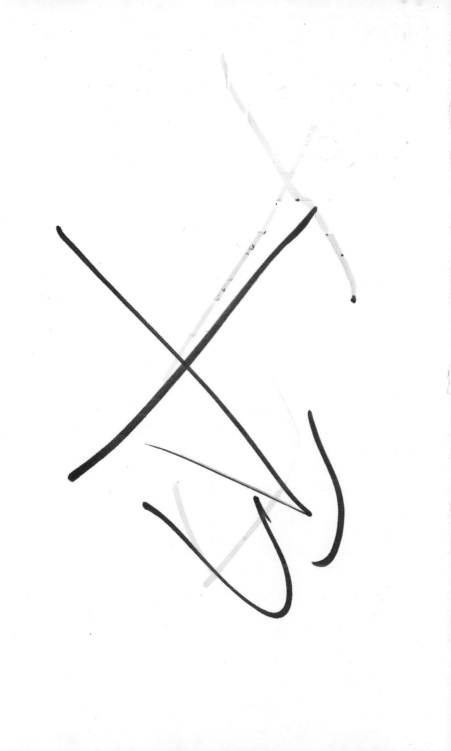